CHEMISTRY OF THE COSMOS

A compilation of writings, epigrams, etc.
—By—

DR. GEO. W. CAREY

TEACHER OF

BIOCHEMISTRY.

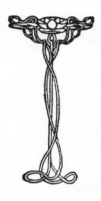

Martino Publishing
Mansfield Centre, CT
2013

Martino Publishing
P.O. Box 373,
Mansfield Centre, CT 06250 USA

ISBN 978-1-61427-460-5

© *2013 Martino Publishing*

Cover design by T. Matarazzo

Printed in the United States of America On 100% Acid-Free Paper

CHEMISTRY OF THE COSMOS

A compilation of writings, epigrams, etc.
—By—

Dr. Geo. W. Carey

TEACHER OF

BIOCHEMISTRY.

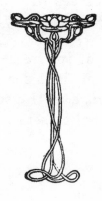

THE LLEWELLYN PUBLISHING CO.
1507 S. Ardmore Ave., Los Angeles, California.

FREEDOM.

The rain that falls in the heart of man,
  Flows out through the eyes in tears;
And God's decrees in the soul of man,
  Are wrought in the cycle of years.

Mortal thought in the heart of man,
  Is flotsam on life's sea
The divine urge in the soul of man
  Is the word that sets him free.

TABLE OF CONTENTS.

"IT," OR THE ETERNITY OF PERFECTION.

By Dr. George W. Carey, Teacher of Biochemistry.

Divine intelligence, the one universal substance, as we unconsciously admit whenever we say, "It rains!" or "It is cold!" All Nature's manifestations due to different vibrations of this one substance, which, by a knowledge of its laws, may be changed and molded to man's will.

A child brought to its mother a piece of ice, and asked: "What is this?"

The mother answered, "It is ice."

Again the child asked, "What is there in ice?"

"There is water in ice," answered the mother.

The child desired to find the water in the ice, and it procured a hammer, and pounded the piece of ice into little bits, and the warm air soon changed all the ice to water. The child was grievously disappointed, for the ice that the child supposed contained water had disappeared.

And the child said, "Where is the ice that contained this water?"

And so it came to pass that the mother was compelled, by the persistent questions, to say, "Ice is all water; there is no such thing as ice; that which we call ice is crystallized or frozen water."

The child understood.

A student brought to his teacher some water and asked, "What is water? What does it contain?"

The teacher answered, "Water contains oxygen and

hydrogen," and then explained how the two gases might be separated and set free by heat.

The student boiled the water until all of the molecules of oxygen and hydrogen had been set free, but he was surprised to find that all of the water had disappeared.

Then the student asked of the teacher, "Where is the water that held the gases that have escaped?"

Then was the teacher compelled by the student's persistent questions to answer, "Water itself is the product of oxygen and hydrogen. Water does not contain anything other than these gases. In reality, there is no such substance or fluid as water; that which we name water is a rate of motion set in operation by the union of two parts of hydrogen with one part of oxygen, and of course the phenomenon disappears when the union of the gases is broken."

The student understood.

A devout scientist presented himself before God and said, "Lord, what are these gases men call oxygen and hydrogen?"

The good Lord answered and said, "They are molecules in the blood and body of the universe."

Then spoke the scientist, "Lord, wilt Thou tell me of the kind of molecules that compose Thy blood and body?"

The Lord replied, "These same molecules, gases, or principles, compose My blood and body; for I and the universe are one and the same."

Once again the scientist said, "My Lord, may I ask, then, what is spirit and what is matter?"

And thus answered the Lord:

"As ice and water are one, and the gases and water are one, so is spirit and matter one. The different phases and manifestations recognized by man in the molecules of My body—that is, the universe—are caused by the Word; thus, they are My thoughts clothed with form."

Now the scientist felt bold, being redeemed from fear, and asked, "Is my blood, then, identical with Thy blood in composition and divine essence?"

And the Lord said, "Yea, thou art one with the Father."

The scientist now understood and said:

"Now mine eyes are opened, and I preceive that when I eat, I partake of Thy body; when I drink, I drink of Thy blood, and when I breathe, I breathe Thy spirit."

So-called matter is Pure Intelligence and nothing else —because there is not anything else.

Pure intelligence cannot progress or become better. There is nothing but Intelligence. Omnipresence, Omnipotence, Omniscience must mean Intelligence; therefore, these terms are all included in the word.

Let us adopt a short word that will express all that the above written words are intended to express, namely: the word IT. "I" stands for all—the eternal I. "T" stands for operation, manifestation, vibration, action or motion. The "I" in motion is "T," or Crossification, viz: the T-cross. We say, "IT rains!" IT is cold!" "IT is all right!" What do we mean by "IT?" Who knows? Some say, "The weather!" Others, "Natural phenomena!" Very well, then—what do we mean by "the weather," or "natural phenomena?" Why, just IT, of course!

IT does not progress; it does not need to. IT forever manifests, operates, differentiates and presents different aspects or viewpoints of ITSELF. But these different phases are neither good, better nor best, neither bad nor worse—simply different shades and colorings of the One and Only Intelligence.

Every so-called thing, whether it be animal, vegetable, or mineral, molecule or atom, ion or electron, is the result of the One Intelligence expressing itself in different rates of motion. Then what is Spirit?

Spirit means breath or life. Spirit, that which is breathed into man, must be Intelligence, or man would not be intelligent. Non-intelligent substance, which is, of course, unthinkable, would not breathe into anything, nor make it intelligent if it did. Therefore we see that Spirit, Intelligence and Matter are one and the same in different rates of motion.

So-called molecules, atoms, electrons, know what to do. They know where and how to cohere, unite and operate to form a leaf or a flower. They know how to separate and disintegrate that same leaf or flower. These particles of omnipresent life build planets, suns and systems; they hurl the comet on its way across measureless desert of star-dust, and emboss its burning trail.

From the materialistic and individual concept of life and its operations, it is pitiable and pathetic to view the wrecks along the shores of science. It is only when we view these apparently sad failures from the firm foothold of the unity of being and the operation of wisdom that we clearly see in these frictions and warring elements and temporary defeats and victories the chemical operation of Eternal Spirit—operating with its own substance—its very self. It is only through the fires of transmutation that we are enabled to see that all life is one Eternal Life and therefore cannot be taken, injured or destroyed.

The fitful, varying, changing beliefs of souls in the transition stage from the sleep and dreams of materialism to the realization of the Oneness of Spirit show forth in a babel of words and theories, a few of which I shall briefly consider, beginning with the yet popular belief in evolution:

The evolutionary concept has its starting point in the idea (a) that matter—so-called—is a something separate from mind, intelligence, or spirit; (b) that this matter had a beginning; (c) that it contains within itself the desire to progress or improve, and finally, that the race is progressing, becoming wiser, better, etc.

Again this assumption, I submit the proposition that the universe—one verse— always existed without beginning or ending, and is and always has been absolutely perfect in all its varied manifestations and operations.

A machine is no stronger than its weakest part. If the self-existing universe is weak or imperfect in any part, it must of necessity, always have been so. Having all the knowledge there is—being all—it is unthinkable that there is any imperfection anywhere. Everything we see, feel, or taste, or in any manner sense, is perfect substance, condensed or manifested from perfect elements, but all differ in their notes, vibrations or modes or rates of motion. A serpent is as perfect, therefore as good, as a man. Without feet, it outruns man; without hands, it outclimbs the ape, and has been à symbol of wisdom through all the ages. Man is an evil thing to the serpent's consciousness as truly as the serpent is an evil thing to the man's consciousness. Neither are evil—nor good. They are different expressions or variations of the "Play of the Infinite Will."

The brain of the jelly-fish is composed of the same elements of the same substance as the brain of a man, merely of a different combination. Can man tell what the jelly-fish is thinking, or why it moves and manifests its energy thus or so? How, then, is man wiser than the jelly-fish because his thoughts are of a different nature, and operate to different ends?

Wisdom—all there is—simply operates, manifests, expresses forms, or creates of itself. As wisdom is without being or end, so are all its operations or manifestations without beginning or end. If the race is constantly evolving to higher standards and loftier conceptions, why send young men and women to Rome and Florence to study the "Old Masters"? If man has evolved up from the "lower forms of life," why has he spent so much time, money and brain energy in trying to understand these lower forms, and to do what they do? Why does he not remember and retain the power of his earlier states of manifestation?

The eagle must wonder, as it watches man's efforts and failures to perfect his flying machine, how long it will be before he evolves up to the science of the birds, i. e., the science of flying. Modern man is now taking his first lessons in condensing air, while through unnumbered ages the spider has performed the miracle without the necessity of first attending a school of chemistry. The modus operandi by which he materializes his web from air is the despair of science. The

wisdom of the ant or beaver strikes dumb all the believers in the Darwinian dream. The perfect co-operative commonwealth of the bees is still the unattainable
ideal of man.

Beneath the soil upon which falls the shadow of the
throne of Menelik, the Abyssinian King, are layers and
strata of buried civilizations, and astronomers in China
mapped the Heavens, named the stars, calculated
eclipses and the return of comets ages before Moses
led the Hebrews out of bondage, or the walls of Balbeck
cast a shade for the Arab and his camel.

The evidences and witnesses of the wisdom of men on
earth hundreds of thousands of years ago confront the
scientific investigator at every turn. Here the Rossetta
Stone, and there the Inscribed Cylinder of Arioch or
Statue of Gudea, King of Chaldea. Prophecies, inscribed on cuniform tablets of clay, foretelling the building of the Pyramids, are brought to light by the excavator: and the history of the Chinese Empire, running
back in links of an unbroken chain for one hundred and
fifty thousand years, forever refute the theory of the
"Descent of Man!" Side by side with the ancient
Asiatics who knew all that we today know, dwelt the
Crystal, the Cell, the Jelly-Fish, the Saurian, the Ape,
and the Cave-Man. Side by side with the masons who
could build arches of stone in ancient Yucatan that
mock at the ravages of time, lived and wrought the ant,
operating in its co-operative commonwealth of which
man can still only dream. Side by side with the cave
men and cannibals dwells the spider whose operation
in aerial elements is the despair of chemical investi-
gators. And when Solomon's golden-spired temple il-
luminated the Holy City, or the Tower of Babel grew

toward the clouds, or the Mound Builders recorded their
history in rock and soil, the eagle and the dove calmly
floated in the air and wondered when men would evolve
to their plane of science. They are wondering still.

Exponents of the evolutionary theory never tire in
quoting Professor Huxley. One who has not read the
writings of this eminent scientist would be led to believe by the statements of his followers that he had
positive views on the great question of force and matter
Following is an extract from a letter written by Professor Huxley to Charles Kingsley under date of May 22,
1863, taken from the published letters of Huxley by his
son, Leonard:

"I don't know whether Matter is anything distinct
from Force. I don't know that atoms are anything but
pure myths—'Cogito ergo sum' is to my mind a ridicu-
lous piece of bad logic, all I can say at any time being
'Cogito.' The Latin form I hold to be preferable to the
English 'I think,' because the latter asserts the existence of an Ego—about which the bundle of phenomena
at present addressing you knows nothing. I believe in
Hamilton, Mansell and Herbert Spencer, so long as they
are destructive, and laugh at their beards as soon as
they try to spin their own cobwebs.

"Is this basis of ignorance broad enough for you? If
you, theologian, can find as firm footing as I, man of
science, do on this foundation of minus naught—there
will be naught to fear for our ever diverging. For
you see, I am quite as ready to admit your doctrine that
souls secrete bodies as I am the opposite one that
bodies secrete souls—simply because I deny the possibility of obtaining any evidence as to the truth or
falsehood of either hypothesis. My fundamental axiom

of speculative philosophy is that materialism and spiritualism are opposite poles of the same absurdity—the absurdity of imagining that we know anything about either spirit or matter."

Huxley admitted that he did not know.

As the appetite craves new chemical combinations of food from day to day, so does mind or soul crave new concepts of infinite life. The word "Infinite" defines an endless differentiation of concept.

If the Spiritual Consciousness—the "mighty Angel" that the clairvoyant seer, John the Revelator, saw descending out of the Heavens, shall carry away the pillars of material evolution, a Temple of Truth divinely fair will spring, Phoenix-like, to take its place. Eyes shall then be opened, and ears unstopped. Man will then realize that the so-called lower forms of life are just as complex, wonderful and difficult to form as the organism of man—that protoplasm is just as wonderful in any other form as in the gray matter of the human brain, which is only another form of its expression—that the molecular composition of a jelly-fish puzzles the greatest chemist, and that the wisdom of a beaver is enough to strike dumb all the believers in the Darwinian fairy tale.

And has the dream of good and evil any better foundation than has this one of material evolution? We are here to solve the problems of life, not to evade them; and to name the mighty operations of Eternal Wisdom good and evil is simply evading instead of solving.

The universal Principle, Spirit, or God, is impartial. Saint and Sinner are one in the Eternal Mind. There is no point in the universe better, higher or nearer

God, or the center, than any other point. All places are necessary, and no one is favored over any other. As Huxley well said, "Good and evil are opposite poles of the same absurdity." Good must have evil for its opposite, if it exists at all. He who would realize being must get rid of the concept of good, as well as the concept of evil. Good and evil are qualifications, and Being does not admit of qualification or graduation. It simply is. The ideal we call good eternally exists, but its name is wisdom's operations. Nothing is low or high, good or bad, except to individual concept that allows comparison. "Comparisons are odious."

Physical Science, so-called, declares in its text-books that light travels from the sun to the earth in eight minutes—a distance of about ninety-five million miles. To question this statement a few years ago meant ostracism from the circle of the elect who knew things. But today the iconoclast stands at the gates of the temples of learning and batters at their walls with the hammer of Thor. Fear and trembling seize upon the votaries of material gods as they see evolution, progression, the theories of electricity, light and heat, good and evil, all cast into the crucible of truth for transmutation in the Divine Alchemy of Being, all dissolving as pieces of ice of different sizes and shapes change to water.

The present day chemist, as he begins to tread the soil where stood the ancient alchemist, tells us that light and heat are simply rates of motion of a substance that does not travel from star to star or from sun to planet, but vibrates in its place at rates directed by the Eternal Word. This substance, aerial or etheric, does not travel—it is everywhere present—the body of omnipresent being.

Men now dare assert that there is no evidence that the sun is hot, but that there is evidence that the sun is the dynamo of the solar system, and so vibrates the etheric substance that light, heat and cold and gravitation are produced—not as entities separate from the universal elements, but as results or effects produced by different rates of motion of the molecules that constitute the body of the universe in their place. The Infinite Word did not command light to go from the sun to the planets, but said, "Let there be light."

We are now told by the remorseless iconoclastic truth-finder that there is no such thing as electricity; that it is a myth so far as fluid or any kind of substance is concerned. The man with the battering ram at the gates of the temple of Maya, or illusion, says that the phenomenon we have named electricity is simply an intensely high rate of vibration, oscillation or motion of the molecules of the wire—molecular motion—or of the air or etheric substance, as in wireless telegraphy.

Another ancient belief, now obsolete, is the progression of soul in a better state of existence after death or cessation of bodily functions. This idea had its origin in the fallacy that there were grades of goodness in the Divine Mind, and that somehow we are not treated right during earth life, and that, in consequence, we must be rewarded by an easy berth "over there." But we now see quite clearly that the great cause of life and all its operations would be unjust to withhold from its sons and daughters for one moment anything that belonged to them. If the Cause ever does wrong, we see no reason why it should repent and do right. If the Cause ever failed in the least particular to give just dues it may do so again at any time.

The time was, and not so very long ago, when the recognized scientists believed that there were about seventy-four elements, indivisible, separate and distinct; but the alchemical iconoclast with his hammer of truth has pulverized the fallacy and remorselessly hammered and pounded the seventy-four faces into one countenance until: "Clothed with the oneness of being, we acknowledge dominion of soul."

For a long time, hydrogen gas, the negative pole of water, was supposed to be indivisible beyond all question; but the present day chemist knows it is only an expression of yet more subtle molecules back of which "Standeth God within the shadow keeping watch above His own."

Between the phantasy of the "Mortal mind" wastebasket, out of which so-called matter forever wriggles to confront the disciples of Berkeley and clamor for recognition, to the Prodigal Son concept of Mental Science that repeats, "All is mnid," "All is good," "I am success," "I attract all that I need," "I am free," "I am health," etc., lies the wrecks of Isms like the thrones and sceptres of kings and rulers along the highway of nations. Mental Science teachers assert that they live in the Universal Opulence—but many can't pay their rent. They declare that they are health —but many times fail to cure their own ailments. How can health get sick or need affirmations? They stoutly maintain that they have absolute control over their bodies, but some of them are five feet two and weigh two hundred pounds. They claim that they are free, but yet they are convicted of violation of law and locked up in prison.

There is no reward in the Eternal plan for doing good or right thinking. Good is relative. We cognize good only by contrast with something unpleasant to us, and that which one calls good, another calls evil. Wisdom proceeds or operates, but does not reward or punish. Wisdom is not personal—it is universal; therefore there is nothing to reward or punish.

A post morten examination of some of the wrecks along the shores of the troubled sea of science discloses a belief that the soul or Ego is an individual, who, through knowledge of its divine origin, may draw unto itself all things it may desire! But as fast as the sleepers awaken, they see that each soul is only "part of one stupendous whole," that does not draw unto itself anything: that there is no law of attraction, for the eternal substance is everywhere present and each one uses exactly that portion prepared for him from everlasting unto everlasting.

When the continuity of life was first demonstrated beyond question, those who caught the first dispatches from disincarnate spirits sprang forth from their beds of material sleep and with half-opened eyes only saw the great truth "as through glass darkly." Then came a babel of words. They jabbered a jargon that needed translation to be understood. The ideas of progression in earth life that obtained among men was translated to the spirit realm, and we were told by the votaries of spiritual philosophy that souls had great opportunities for progression after leaving the flesh. As the idea of a commencement of the universe was a common belief among souls asleep in material consciousness, being the cornerstone of evolution, so the idea was taught that the individual had a commencement in the maternal human laboratory. As these half-awakened souls could not comprehend that an action contrary to their concept of good could possibly be caused by Infinite Intelligence, they concluded that the so-called bad actions of men and women were prompted by evil earth-bound spirits. These people—many of them—also thought that the main object of the existence of spirits in the Spirit Realm was to gather information about mines, and stocks, and bonds, and lotteries, and races, and thus assist poor mortals to get rich quick. It was supposed that these spirits were posted in regard to deeds and wills and knew when wealthy relatives would shuffle off this mortal coil, or when undesirable wives or husbands would "pass out."

But at last the Sun of Truth pierced the darkness and the jargon of selfishness changed to the "New Song." We now clearly see that each spirit is a part or attribute of the One Eternal Spirit—therefore has always existed; and that the process of generation deals with flesh clothing, or mask for the spirit, in which it performs a necessary part in the creative process. The word "person" is derived from a Greek word meaning mask. We see that the phenomena we have called obsession by evil spirits is God's surgery or dynamic operation in His own temple, quite as impossible for us to understand in our present environment as it is for the child to understand the wisdom and necessity in the operation of the adept surgeon. And, finally, we now see and fully realize that Eternal Wisdom, without beginning or end of days, does not progress before entering a temple of flesh, nor while it occupies it, nor after it leaves it. All creative or formative processes may properly be termed operations of wisdom, or Eternal Life.

In the unwalled temple of the Now, beneath its roofless dome, lighted by myriad suns, there is neither beginning nor end: neither good nor evil. Within the domain of this necessity, there is no evolution from low to high. There is nothing low. Within the realm of being there is no progression, but a constantly moving panorama forever presenting to consciousness new phases of the absolute.

The men and women who do things take hold of the opportunities and material that they find all about them now, and operate with them, astonishing results following the efforts of all who recognize that eternal force has use for men NOW to carry out the divine plan. We are all operators or workmen in the divine workshop, and the Divine Intelligence, the eternal IT, made no mistake in placing any of us here, but does insist that we recognize that Now is the time and Here is the place to do our best. As the Great Cause does not need to first practice on lower forms in order at some future time to attain perfection, we must recognize and practice being in the present, instead of becoming in the future, for the Eternal Now is all the time there is.

"But," you say, "your science has taken away my God, and I know not where you have lain Him." On the contrary, I have brought you to the one true God, "which was, and is, and evermore shall be."

The fifth verse of the last chapter of the book of Job reads as follows:

"I have heard of thee by the hearing of mine ear; but now mine eye seeth thee."

The wonderful writings and scientific statements found in that Book of all books, the Christian Bible, were recorded at dates covering thousands of years by men and women who never heard of each other. Some of these teachers lived away back in the age when the solar system was swinging through the zodiacal sign Taurus; when Phallic worship prevailed; when the number six was understood as sex, and the creative or formative principle operating through the sex functions was worshiped as the very Holy of Holies. Other teachers who contributed to the knowledge of life and its operations contained in the Bible, lived in the age of Aries, a fire sign, when fire and sun were worshiped as the very essence of good; and as heat, the cause of the phenomenon called fire, cannot be seen, it was a reasonable thing to say that "no one can see God and live." So, then, it depends upon the point of view one has of God, or the spirit of things, whether he says, "No one can see God and live," or says, "Now mine eye seeth thee!"

I think the writer of the book named Job must have lived more than eight thousand years ago, even before the Taurian age—symbolized by the Winged Bull of Nineveh—which was in the Gemini age, the age of perception and expression, being an air age. Let it be understood that an age in this connection means twenty-two hundred years, the period for the sun to pass across one of the signs of the zodiac. In an air age, souls awaken to their divine heritage, and realize their God-hood. The writer of Job, then, living in the Gemini or air age, could see God and live. Our solar system has entered the sign Aquarius, another air sign, and the spiritualized elements so act upon our brain cells that we are able to understand the teachers of a past air age, and also see God and live.

Carlyle, the prince of literary critics, said, "The book of Job is the most wonderful and beautiful literary production ever given to the world." Certainly the scientific truths of astrology and alchemy, and of the soul's operation in flesh, as set forth in that book, are without a parallel. The letters J O B have an occult, scientific meaning, I and J are the same, IOB meaning the same as JOB. I means the eternal I. All the Hebrew letters were formed from I. O means the universe, without beginning or end, and B means Beth, a body, house, church, or temple. Therefore GOD, or all, may be discovered as seen in JOB or IOB. The word Job has no reference to a person. The name, or letters of the word, symbolize principle, the same as wisdom, knowledge, intelligence, or Christ, or Buddha. We symbolize the principles of our government in personalities, and picture them in the form of a man or woman, namely Uncle Sam, or Columbia. But we do more than that—we put words in their mouth, and make them utter speech. And shall we ignore these facts when dealing with the record of past ages? One record plainly states that Jesus spake only in parables.

But let us consider more closely the discovery of God. The numerical value of GOD, according to ancient Kabala, is nine—the all of mathematics—no person is alluded to. If the statement, "I and the Father are one," is true, the "I" must be the Father manifested or expressed. As it is not possible to conceive of the Father except through expression, we must conclude that manifestation in some form of so-called matter is eternal—the great necessity—and has therefore always been.

It is quite reasonable to think that some oxygen and hydrogen has eternally existed in gaseous form, some in the combination that causes water and some in the more concrete or concentrated form known as ice. Then upon the postulate that Spirit and matter—that is, bodily or material expression—are one, it follows logically that matter, including the physical body or temple or man, is as necessary to the Father-Mother principle while held in a given rate of activity or expression as this life essence is necessary to matter, or the physical structure of man. I see oxygen and hydrogen when I look at the manifestation we call ice. When I see water, I know just how oxygen and hydrogen appear when united. So when I look at any form of so-called matter, I know exactly how GOD appears at that particular time and place. I do not see the effect or works of God, but I see God, and just as much of God, face to face, as I am capable of seeing or recognizing at a certain time.

Step by step, the scientific investigator is being led to the threshold of the awful, absolute TRUTH, that all matter, or substance, or energy or force—call it what you may—is not only intelligent, but is Pure Intelligence itself. Atoms, molecules, electrons, are but expressions of rates of motion of pure Mind, Thought, or Intelligence that man has personified and called God. Ice is not permeated with water, or controlled by water. Ice is water. Matter is not controlled by mind; mind and matter are one. A high vibration of mind does control, to a certain extent, a lower vibration of mind, as water may carry a lump of ice here or there, water being a more positive rate of activity of the same thing. The particles, so-called, of matter know what to do. The atoms that compose a leaf know when to cohere and materialize a leaf, and they know when to disintegrate and dematerialize it: "Thou shalt have no other gods."

I hold in my hand that particular form of the one thing called a rose. Material thought says it is made by God, or that God is in the rose or back of it, or that God caused or created it; but when Spirit asks where is the God that created the rose, where He has betaken Himself, material belief is silent. But hold a moment! I have here a bud, a half-formed rose. If God makes a rose, He must continue the work to completion. Ah, speak softly! Look closely! The rose is now being made, and you say God is making it. Yes, you said God made this full-blown rose. Bring on your spectroscope, your microscope! Quick, now, you chemist! Bring on your test-tubes, your acids, and alkalis! Analyze, illuminate, and magnify! Now we shall discover God. He is here at work before your eyes.

What do you see, chemist? What do you see, scientist? Ah! I know what you see. My experience in the realm of matter and of Spirit tell me what you see. O thou stupendous sex force—sex—days of creation, thou Father-Mother Yahveh, thou divine male and female, thou eternal positive and negative dynamis! We now behold thee operating. Out from the chemicalizing mass of God's creative compounds, out of the quivering, vibrating substance, slowly comes forth the rose. But are you sure it is a rose? Hold a moment. What is a rose? Of what material is it formed? Ah! the chemist speaks—he of the crucibles and test-tubes and acids! Hear the chemist!

He says, "The rose is made from the universal substance," or "The rose is universal substance, in a certain rate of activity." Thanks! Blessed be the chemist! Universal—one verse—one substance—no other substance—God is the rose, or the smile we call a rose —God is again manifested in the great Eternal IT, for which there is no other name.

> "Acids and alkalis acting,
>   Proceeding and acting again,
> Operating, transmuting, fomenting,
>   In throes and spasms of pain—
> Uniting, reacting, atoning,
>   Like souls passing under the rod—
> Some people call it Chemistry,
>   Others call it GOD."

Job did not say, "I see the thoughts of God," nor did he say, "I can fathom the mind of God." The plan cannot be seen; but that which is planned—a planet— can be seen. One may see the substance of God without understanding the mind of God.

Let us hear Emerson on this stupendous, glorious theme:

> "The great Idea baffles wit;
>   Language falters under it;
>   It leaves the learned in the lurch—
>   Nor art, nor power, nor toil can find
>   The measure of the Eternal Mind,
>   Nor hymn, nor prayer, nor church."

O thou ever-present Divine Mind and Substance! We now fully realize our oneness with thee, and bathe and revel in thy glory. The mighty Angel of Reality has torn the veil of illusion, and we see the celestial City of Truth with wide open gates and the white light of Eternal Love forever upon its streets.

O soul, in the shadow of sickness and trial, "Take up thy bed and walk; thy sins be forgiven thee."

"ARMAGEDDON" AND ASTROLOGY.

By Dr. Geo. W. Carey, Teacher of Biochemistry.

One of the so-called strong points used by the opponents of Astrology is the fact that 50,000 soldiers are sometimes killed in one battle.

Our skeptical friends say that according to Astrology no person dies except there be a planetary combination that indicates death at that particular time. But our critics are not aware of the fact that the Astrologers of Europe have for the past ten years or more remarked the similarity of planetary aspects in the "House of Death" of a large proportion of nativities examined.

This startling fact was clearly established in the wreck of the Titanic. Every person lost on that ill-starred boat, so far as data has been secured in regard to their birth, had planetary combinations indicating death at that time. Those who escaped were under aspects that indicated danger of drowning, but at the same time had a favorable aspect of Jupiter or Venus or both.

Another proof that Astrology, Physiology and Chemistry are all links in the chain of life, the eternal sequence of things and events, I cite the fact that the great palmists of Europe have declared for many years that there must be some great catyclism near, as the fate line in a large majority of hands terminated suddenly.

If the above be true, and I believe that it is true, it opens up a wide field of biochemical research. For it is quite evident to all students of Biochemistry that the cell-salts of the blood are the tissue builders; therefore the lines in the hand are formed by the chemical operation of these workers through the blood.

And so it may yet come to pass that by the analysis of blood, the use of the Spectroscope, the Cathode ray, the physiologist may be enabled to foretell accidents or death and thus rule his stars through wisdom.

Biochemistry may be called Astrology in solution, and when the chemists, electricians and other scientists of the world turn their attention to this deeply fascinating study, it may be that man will learn to so place the positive and negative poles of being that he can produce forms of life at will. And more, man may by the study of the great machine, the universe of which he is an integral part, so construct, build and create that he will bring forth forms from the "Universal energy from which all things proceed" under favorable planetary positions that will make for harmony and peace instead of discord and war.

When conception and birth are scientifically understood on the higher intellectual plane, animalism will be transmitted into spiritual understanding and the age of man commence its reign on earth.

THE WONDERS AND POSSIBILITIES OF THE HUMAN BODY.

The human race has been asleep, and has dreamed that property and money are the true wealth of a nation, sacrificing men, women and children to the chimerical idea that danced in visionary splendor through their brains. The result of this is to be seen in the uneasiness that prevails everywhere. But humanity is waking up, slowly but surely, and beginning to realize that it, itself, is the most precious thing on earth.

The old-established statement that the individuals that make up the race are imperfect is no more true than that a pile of lumber is imperfect, that is to be afterward reformed, or built into a house. As it is the carpenter's business to take the lumber, which is perfect as material, and build the house, so it is the legitimate work of spiritual man to take the perfect material everywhere present and build, by the perfect law of chemistry and mathematics, the perfected, harmonious human being, and with this material, employ the same law to build up society collectively.

It is a well-known physiological fact that the blood is the basic material of which the human body is continually builded. As is the blood, so is the body; as is the body, so is the brain; as is the brain, so is the quality of thought. As a man is builded, so thinks he.

According to the views of students of modern alchemy, the Bible—both the Old and New Testaments—are symbolical writings, based primarily upon this very process of body building. The word Alchemy really means Fleshology. It is derived from Chem, an ancient Egyptian word, meaning flesh. The word Egypt also means flesh, or anatomy.

Alchemy, however, in its broader scope, means the science of solar rays. Gold may be traced to the Sun's rays. The word gold means solar essence. The transmutation of gold does not mean the process of making gold, but does mean the process of changing gold, solar rays, into all manner of materialized forms, vegetable, mineral, etc. The ancient alchemist studied the process of Nature in her operations from the volatile to the fixed, the fluid to the solid, the essence to the substance, or the abstract to the concrete, all of which may be summed up in the changing of spirit into matter. In reality, the alchemist did not try to do anything. He simply tried to search out nature's processes in order that he might comprehend her marvelous operations.

To be sure, language was used that to us seems symbolical and often contradictory, but it was not so intended, nor so at all in reality. We speak in symbols. If a man is in delirium, caused by alcohol in his brain-cells, we say he has "snakes in his boots." Of course, no one supposes that the words are to be taken literally. Yet if our civilization should be wiped out, and our literature translated after four or five thousand years, those who read our history might be puzzled to know what was meant by "snakes in his boots."

Again, it has been believed by most people that the words, "transmutation of base metals into gold," used by alchemists, referred to making gold. But a careful study of the Hebrew Cosmogony, and the Kabala, will reveal the fact that the alchemist always referred to solar rays when he used the word gold. By "base metals," they simply meant matter, or basic. The dissolving or disintegration of matter, the combustion of wood or coal, seemed as wonderful to these philosophers as the growth of wood or the formation of coal or stone. So, the transmutation of base metals into gold simply meant the process of changing the fixed into the volatile, or the dematerialization of matter, either by heat or chemical process.

It is believed by modern students of alchemy that the books of the Old and New Testaments are a collection of alchemical and astrological writings, dealing entirely with the wonderful operation of aerial elements (Spirit) in the human body, so fearfully and wonderfully made. The same authority is given for the statements, "Know ye not that your bodies are the temple of the living God" and "Come unto Me all ye that labor and are heavy laden and I will give ye rest." According to the method of reading the numerical value of letters by the Kabala, M and E figure B, when united. Our B is from the Hebrew Beth, meaning a house or temple—the temple of the soul—the body. Thus by coming into the realization that the body is really the Father's House, temple of God, the soul secures peace and contentment or rest.

The human body is composed of perfect principles, gases, minerals, molecules, or atoms; but these builders, of flesh and bone are not always properly adjusted. The planks or bricks used in building houses may be endlessly diversified in arrangement, and yet be perfect material.

Solomon's temple is an allegory of man's temple—

the human organism. This house is built (always being built) "without sound of saw or hammer."

The real Ego manifests in a house, beth, church, or temple—i. e., Soul-of-Man's Temple.

The solar (soular) plexus is the great central Sun or dynamo on which the Subconscious Mind (another name for God) operates and causes the concept of individual consciousness. The brain of man is the Son of God, the mediator (medium) between the central dynamo and the Cosmic Ocean of Space. Thus digestion or combustion of food, circulation of blood, inbreathing the breath of life, (aerial elements) is carried on by the co-operation of the Holy Trinity; God, the solar plexus; the Son, the brain; and the Holy (whole) Spirit, or air.

No wonder that the seers and alchemists of old declared that "Your bodies are the temple of the living God" and "The kingdom of Heaven is within you." But man, blinded by selfishness, searches here and there, scours the heavens with his telescope, digs deep into earth, and dives into ocean's depths, in a vain search for the Elixir of Life that may be found between the soles of his feet and the crown of his head. Really our human body is a miracle of mechanism. No work of man can compare with it in accuracy of its process and the simplicity of its laws.

At maturity, the human skeleton contains about 165 bones, so delicately and perfectly adjusted that science has despaired of ever imitating it. The muscles are about 500 in number; length of alimentary canal, 32 feet; amount of blood in everage adult, 30 pounds, or one-fifth the weight of the body; the heart is six inches in length and four inches in diameter, and beats seventy times per minute, 4200 times per hour, 100,800 per day, 36,720,000 per year. At each beat, two and one-half ounces of blood are thrown out of it, 175 ounces per minute, 656 pounds per hour, or about eight tons per day.

All the blood in the body passes through the heart every three minutes; and during seventy years it lifts 270,000,000 tons of blood.

The lungs contain about one gallon of air at their usual degree of inflation. We breathe, on an average, 1200 breaths per hour; inhale 600 gallons of air, or 24,000 gallons daily.

The aggregate surface of air-cells of the lungs exceed 20,000 square inches, an area nearly equal to that of a room twelve feet square. The average weight of the brain of an adult is three pounds, eight ounces; the average female brain, two pounds, four ounces. The convolutions of a woman's brain cells and tissues are finer and more delicate in fibre and mechanism, which evidently accounts for the intuition of women. It would appear that the difference in the convolutions and fineness of tissue in brain matter is responsible for the degrees of consciousness called reason and intuition.

The nerves are all connected with the brain directly, or by the spinal marrow, but nerves receive their sustenance from the blood, and their motive power from the solar plexus dynamo. The nerves, together with the branches and minute ramifications, probably ex-

ceed ten millions in numbers, forming a bodyguard out-
numbering the mightiest army ever marshalled.

The skin is composed of three layers, and varies from
one-eighth to one-quarter of an inch in thickness. The
average area of skin is estimated to be about 2000
square inches. The atmospheric pressure, being fourteen pounds to the square inch, a person of medium size
is subject to a pressure of 40,000 pounds. Each square
inch of skin contains 3500 sweat tubes, or perspiratory
pores (each of which may be likened to a little drain
tile) one-fourth of an inch in length, making an aggregate length of the entire surface of the oody 201,166
feet, or a tile for draining the body nearly forty miles
in length.

Our body takes in an average of five and a half pounds
of food and drink each day, which amounts to one ton
of solid and liquid nourishment annually, so that in
seventy years a man eats and drinks 1000 times his
own weight.

There is not known in all the realms of architecture
or mechanics one little device which is not found in
the human organism. The pulley, the lever, the in-
clined plane, the hinge, the "universal joint" tubes and
trap-doors; the scissors, grind-stone, whip, arch, girders,
filters, valves, bellows, pump, camera, and Aeolian harp;
and irrigation plant, telegraph and telephone systems—
all these and a hundred other devices which man thinks
he has invented, but which have only been telegraphed
to the brain from the Solar Plexus (cosmic centre)
and crudely copied or manifested on the objective canvas.

No arch ever made by man is as perfect as the arch formed by the upper ends of the two legs and the pelvis to support the weight of the trunk. No palace or cathedral ever built has been provided with such a perfect system of arches and girders.

No waterway on earth is so complete, so commodious, or so populous as that wonderful river of life, the "Stream of Blood." The violin, the trumpet, the harp, the grand organ, and all the other musical instruments, are mere counterfeits of the human voice.

Man has tried in vain to duplicate the hinges of knee, elbow, fingers and toes, although they are a part of his own body.

Another marvel of the human body is the self-regulation process by which nature keeps the temperature in health at 98 degrees. Whether in India, with the temperature at 130 degrees, or in the arctic regions, where the records show 120 degrees below the freezing point, the temperature of the body remains the same, practically steady at 98 degrees, despite the extreme to which it is subjected.

It was said that "all roads lead to Rome." Modern science has discovered that all roads of real knowledge lead to the human body. The human body is an epitome of the universe; and when man turns the mighty searchings of reason and investigation within that he has so long used without—the New Heaven and Earth will appear.

While it is true that flesh is made by a precipitation of blood, it is not true that blood is made from food.

The inorganic or cell-salts contained in food are set free by the process of combustion or digestion, and carried into the circulation through the delicate absorbent tubes of the mucous membrane of stomach and intestines. Air, or Spirit, breathed into the lungs, enters the arteries (air carriers) and chemically unites with the mineral base, and by a wonderful transformation creates flesh, bone, hair, nails, and all the fluids of the body.

On the rock (Peter or Petra, meaning stone) of the mineral salts is the human structure built, and the grave, stomach, or hell shall not prevail against it. The minerals in the body do not disintegrate or rot in the grave.

The fats, albumen, fibrine, etc., that compose the organic part of food, are burned up in the process of digestion and transposed into energy or force to run the human battery. Blood is made from air; thus all nations that dwell on earth are of one blood, for all breathe one air. The best food is the food that burns up quickest and easiest; that is, with the least friction in the human furnace.

The sexual functions of man and woman; the holy operation of creative energy manifested in male and female; the formation of life germs in ovum and sex fluids; the Divine Procedure of the "word made flesh" and the mysteries of conception and birth are the despair of science.

"Know ye not that your bodies are the temple of the living God?" for "God breathed into man the breath of life."

In the words of Epictitus, "Unhappy man, thou bear-
est a god with thee, and knows it not."

Walt Whitman sings:

"I loaf and invite my soul; I lean and loaf at my
ease, observing a spear of summer grass. Clear and
sweet is my soul, and clear and sweet is all that is
not my soul."

"Welcome every organ and attribute of me, and of
any man hearty and clean, not an inch, not a particle
of an inch, is vile, and none shall be less familiar than
the rest."

"Divine am I, inside and out, and I make holy whatever I touch or am touched from."

"I say no man has ever yet been half devout enough;
none has ever yet adored or worshipped half enough;
none has begun to think how divine he himself is, and
how certain the future is."

The vagus nerve, so named because of its wandering
(vagrant) branches, is the greatest marvel of the human organism. Grief depresses the circulation, through
the vagus, a condition of malnutrition follows, and tuber-
culosis, often of the hasty type, follows.

The roots of the vagus nerve are in the medulla
oblongata, at the base of the small brain or cerebellum,
and explains why death follows the severing of the

medulla. It controls the heart action, and if a drug such as aconite be administered, even in small doses, its effect upon this nerve is shown in slowing the action of the heart and decreasing the blood pressure. In larger doses it paralyzes the ends of the vagus in the heart, so that the pulse becomes suddenly very rapid and at the same time irregular. Branches of the vagus nerve reach the heart, lungs, stomach, liver and kidneys.

Worry brings on kidney disease, but it is the vagus nerve, and especially that branch running to the kidneys which under undue excitement or worry, or strain, brings about the paralysis of the kidneys in the performance of their functions.

When we say that a man's heart sinks within him for fear or apprehension, it is shown by the effect of this nerve upon the heart action. If his heart beats high with hopes, or he sighs for relief, it is the vagus nerve that has conducted the mental state to the heart and accelerated its action or caused that spasmodic action of the lungs which we call a sigh.

The nerves of the human body constitute the "Tree of Life," with its leaves of healing. The flowing waters of the Rivers of Life are the veins and arteries through which sweep the red, magnetic currents of Love—of Spirit made visible.

Behold the divine telegraph system, the million nerve wires running throughout the wondrous temple, the temple not made with hands, the temple made "without sound of saw or hammer." View the Central Sun of the human system—the Solar Plexus—vibrating life abundantly.

Around this dynamo of God, you may see the Beasts that worship before the Throne day and night saying, "Holy, holy, art Thou, Lord God Almighty." The Beasts are the twelve plexuses of nerve centers, telegraph stations, like unto the twelve zodiacal signs that join hands in a fraternal circle across the gulf of space.

Aviation, liquified air, deep breathing for physical development and the healing of divers diseases rule the day. In every brain there are dormant cells, waiting for the "coming" of the bridegroom, the vibration of the air age (the Christ) that will resurrect them

Everywhere we have evidence of the awakening of dormant brain cells. Much, if not all, of spiritual phenomena, multiple personality, mental telepathy, and kindred manifestations, are explainable upon the hypothesis of the possibility of awakening and bringing into use of dormant- brain cells.

The eye is hardly less wonderful, being a perfect photographer's camera. The retina is the dry plate on which are focused all objects by means of the crystalline lens. The cavity behind this lens is the shutter. The eyelid is the drop shuttle. The draping of the optical dark room is the only black membrane in the entire body. This miniature camera is self-focusing, self-loading and self-developing, and takes millions of pictures every day in colors and enlarged to life size.

Charts have been prepared—marvelous charts—which

go to show that the eye has 729 distinct expressions conveying us many distinct shades of meaning.

The power of color perception is overwhelming. To perceive red the retina of the eye must receive 395,000 vibrations in a second; for violet it must respond to 790,000,000. In our waking moments our eyes are bombarded every minute by at least 600,000,000 vibrations.

The ear is a colossal mystery, and the phenomenon of sound is a secret only recorded in the Holy of Holies of the Infinite Mind. And what is mind? We know absolutely nothing about it. Some believe that mind is the product of the chemical operation of matter, viz.: the atoms or materials that compose the human body. These persons contend that all electrons are particles of pure Intelligence and KNOW what to do. Others hold to the theory that universal Mind (whatever it may be) forms a body from some material, they know not what, and then plays upon it or operates through it.

Visions of beauty and splendor,
   Forms of a long-lost race,
Sounds of faces and voices
   From the fourth dimension of space;
And on through the universe boundless,
   Our thoughts go, lightning-shod;
Some call it Imagination,
   And others call it God!

And last, but not least, comes Speech, the Word that was in the beginning. God certainly bankrupted His infinite series of miracles when He gave the power of speech to man.

We wonder and adore in the presence of that pulsing orb, the heart. Tons of the water of life made red by the Chemistry of Love sweep through this central throne every day, and flow on to enrich the Edenic Garden until its waste places shall bloom and blossom as the rose.

Take my hand and go with me to the home of the Soul—that wondrous brain. Can you count the whirling, electric, vibrating cells? No, not until you can count the sand grains on the ocean's shore. These rainbow-hued cells are the keys that the fingers of the soul strike to play its part in the Symphony of the Spheres.

At last we have seen the "Travail of the Soul and are satisfied." No more temples of the Magi now, but instead the Temple of the Soul, the glorious human Beth. At last we have found the true church of God, the human body. In this body, or church, spirit operates like some wizard chemist or electrician. No more searching through India's jungles or scaling the Himalayan heights in search for a master—a mahatma—or ancient priest dwelling in some mysterious cave where occult rites and ceremonies are supposed to reveal the wisdom of the past. But instead, you have found the Kingdom of the Real within the Temple that needs no outer Sun by day nor Moon nor Stars by night to lighten it. And then the enraptured Soul becomes conscious that the stone has been rolled away from the door of material concept where it has slept, and it now hears the voice of the Father within saying, "Let there be light!" and feels the freedom that comes with knowing that Being is one.

And now Soul also realizes the meaning of the "Day

of Judgment." It realizes that Judgment means understanding, hence the ability to judge. The Soul then judges correctly, for it sees the Wisdom of Infinite Life in all men, in all things, all events, and all environments. Thus does the new birth take place, and the Kingdom of Harmony reigns now.

Man must realize, however, that he is the creator or builder of his own body, and that he is responsible for every moment of its building, and every hour of its care. He alone can select and put together the materials provided by the universe for its construction. Man has been able to scale the heavens, to measure the distances between the stars and planetary bodies, and to analyze the component parts of suns and worlds, yet he cannot eat without making himself ill; he can foretell eclipses and tides for years in advance, but cannot look far enough ahead in his own affairs to say when he may be brought down with la grippe, or to calculate accurately the end of any bodily ill that may afflict him. When he finds out what he really is, and how much he has always had to do in the making of himself what he is, he will be ready to grasp some idea of the wonderful possibilities of every human soul and body, and will know how completely and entirely is every man his own savior. Just so long as he denies his own powers, and looks outside of himself for salvation from present or future ills, he is indeed a lost creature. If the race is to be redeemed, it must come as the result of thought followed by action. If the race is to think differently than at present, it must have new bodies with new brains.

Modern physiologists know that our bodies are completely made over every year, by the throwing off of worn-out cells and the formation of new ones, that is going on every minute. Nature will take care of the making-over process, but we are responsible for the plan of reconstruction. Man must learn to run the machinery of his body with the same mathematical accuracy as he now displays in control of an engine or automobile, before he can lay claim to his divine heritage and proclaim himself master of his own.

The law of life is not a separate agent working independently of mankind and separate from indivdual life. Man himself is a phase of the great law in operation. When he once fully awakens to the universal co-operation of the attributes and thoughts through which the great dynamis operates or proceeds, he—a soul—one of the expressions of infinity, will be enabled to free himself from the seeming environments of matter, and thus realizing his power, will assert his dominion over all he has been an agent in creating. And he has indeed assisted in creating—manifestng—all that is. Being a thought, an outbreathing of universal spirit, he is co-eternal with it.

In material concept, we do not begin to realize the extent of our wisdom. When we awaken to soul, or spirit, consciousness—knowledge that we are souls that have bodies or temples, and not bodies that have souls— we see the object or reason of all symbols or manifestation, and begin to realize our own power over all created things.

And in this Aquarian age, great changes in nature's laws will be speedily brought to pass, and great changes in the affairs of humanity will result. The laws of vibration will be mastered, and through their operation material manifestations will be shaped and moulded to man's will. It is only a matter of time when all the necessities of life will be produced directly from the elements of the air.

It is well known by chemists that all manner of fruits, grains and vegetables are produced directly from the elements in air, and not from soil. The earth, of course, serves as a negative pole and furnishes the mineral salts of lime, magnesium, iron, potassium, sodium and silica, which act as carriers of water, oil, fibrin, sugar, etc., and thus build up the plant; but oil, sugar, albumen, etc., are formed by a precipitation or condensation of principles in air, and not from soil. This is a fact abundantly proved. Mr. Berthelot, a scientist of France, Tesla, the Austrian wizard, and our own Edison have long held that food can be produced by a synthetic process from its elements artificially.

Some six or seven extracts, as well as coloring material, are now being manufactured in this manner. Madder is made almost exclusively by this process now.

Mr. Berthelot, at one time the French minister of foreign affairs, possesses fame apart altogether from his political efforts. In his special domain of chemical knowledge he ranks among the first of his contemporaries. Chemical synthesis—the science of artificially putting organized bodies together—may be said to owe its existence to him. The practical results expected to flow from his experiments and discoveries are enormous. Thus, sugar has recently been made in the laboratory from glycerin, which Professor Berthelot first made direct from synthetic alcohol. Commerce has now taken up the question; and an invention has recently been patented by which sugar is to be made upon a commercial scale, from two gases, at something like 1 cent per pound. M. Berthelot declares he has not the slightest doubt that sugar will eventually be manufactured on a large scale synthetically, and that the culture of sugar cane and beet root will be abandoned, because they have ceased to pay.

The chemical advantages promised by M. Berthelot to future generations are marvelous. He cites the case of alzarin, a compound whose synthetic manufacture by chemists has destroyed a great agricultural industry. It is the essential commercial principle of the madder root, which was once used in dyeing, wherever any dyeing was going on. The chemists have now succeeded in making pure indigo direct from its elements, and it will soon be a commercial product. Then the indigo field, like the madder fields, will be abandoned, industrial laboratories having usurped their place.

But these scientific wonders do not stop here. Tobacco, tea and coffee are to be made artificially; not only this, but there is substantial promise that such tobacco, such teas and such coffees as the world has never seen will be the outcome. Theobromine, the essential principle of the cocoa, has been produced in the laboratory, thus synthetic chemistry is getting ready to furnish the three great non-alcoholic beverages now in general use.

Biochemists long ago advanced the theory that ani-

mal tissue is formed from the air inhaled, and not from
food. The food, of course, serves its purpose; it acts
as the negative pole, as does the earth to plant and
vegetable life, and also furnishes the inorganic salts,
the workers that carry on the chemistry of life, set-
ting free magnetism, heat and electric forces by disintegration and fermentation of the organic portions of
the food.

But air, in passing through the various avenues and
complex structure of the human organism, changes, con-
denses, solidifies, until it is finally deposited as flesh
and bone. From this established scientific truth, it
appears that, by constructing a set of tubes, pumps, etc.,
resembling the circulatory system, as well as the lung
cells of the human mechanism, which is a chemical
laboratory, where the chemistry of spirit is ever at
work, changing the one essence of spirit substance to
blood, flesh and bone, air may be changed into an
albuminous pabulum, which may be again changed into
the special kind of food required by adding the proper
flavor, which may also be produced direct from the air.

There does not seem to be any reason why this substance, the basis of all food or vegetable growth, cannot,
by drying and proper process, be made into material for
clothing. Wool, cotton, flax, silks, etc., are all produced from the universal elements through the slow,
laborious and costly process of animal or vegetable
growth. Why not produce them direct?

Those who believe in a time of peace on earth, a
millennial reign, certainly do not think that our present mode of producing food will continue during that

age. Slaughter of animals, and fruit, grain or vegetable raising leave small time for men and women to
enjoy a condition foretold by all the seers and prophets.
But under the new way of producing food and clothing,
the millennium is possible.

And thus will the problem of subsistence be solved.
No more monopoly of nature's bounties. An exchange
of service will be the coin of the world instead of certain metals difficult to obtain.

When Jesus of Mazereth broke bread and poured wine
(some kind of fluid for drink), we see why He said:
"This is my flesh and blood." He was an adept. He
had spent several years in Egypt and India, and was
aware that all food came from the body of God, universal substance, the one "whose body Nature is, and
God and soul." A realization of this vision, or theory,
that will for awhile be called visionary by most people,
will mean Eden restored. The Earth will be allowed
to return to its natural state. We will cease to eat
animals, birds and fishes, and they will become our
friends, instead of our enemies; love will rule and
break down every barrier. Animals and birds will sub-
sist on the natural products of the soil, as they do in
regions uninhabited by man, with "none to molest
and make them afraid." Many people have wondered
why, during the last few years, fruit pests have multi-
plied so alarmingly, and why cows are almost universally diseased and so much attention given to meat, milk,
and butter products by Boards of Health, etc. There
is surely a reason for all this. The One Life, Supreme
Intelligence, or Divine Wisdom, that holds the worlds
of space in their appointed orbits, surely knows all about

the affairs of earth. When a new dispensation is about
to be ushered in, old things begin to pass away.

All labor of preparing food and clothing, as now
carried on, will cease, and the people, in governmental
or collective capacity, will manufacture and distribute
all manner of food and clothing free. Machinery for the
production of everything necessary for man's material
wants will be simple and easily manipulated. One-
twentieth of the able-bodied population, working one or
two hours a day, and shifting every week, or day, for
that matter, with others, will produce an abundant
supply. Neither droughts nor floods nor winter's snow
can affect the supply. It can be made in Klondyke or
the Tropics. Garments may be worn for a few days and
then burned, and laundry work cease. Cooking will
be reduced to a minimum, as the food will only need
flavoring. No preparing vegetables, fruits, or cracking
nuts; no making butter, or preserving meats. Men will
not have to devote their lives to the endless grind of
food production, nor woman to cooking, dish-washing,
sewing, and laundry-work. Garments of beautiful design
and finest texture will be made by machines invented
for the purpose, ready for wear.

A dream, you say? I cannot admit that in the face of
the indisputable evidence it has already been able to
produce, but what if it were, at present, but the dream
it may appear to the one who hears of its methods
of operation for the first time? Do dreams ever come
true? Yea, verily! All concrete facts are materialized
dreams.

An Egyptian King dreamed, and the Pyramids of

Cheops mass and miracle his vision. The Pyramids are enclopedic of physical science and astral lore. The science of numbers, weights, measures, geometry astronomy, astrology, and all the deeper mysteries of the human body and soul are symboled in these incomparable monuments.

A dream of an ancient alchemist solidified in stone, and the awful sphinx sat down in Egypt's sand to gaze into eternity.

Columbus dreamed, and a white-sailed ship turned its prow west and west. On uncharted seas, with an eternity of water ahead, he remembered his dream, and answered "Sail on!" to the discouraged mate, until he landed on the unknown shores of a most wonderful new world.

Michael Angelo dreamed a thousand dreams and sleeping marble awoke and smiled. Hudson and Fulton dreamed, and steamboats "run over and under the seas."

The Pilgrim Fathers dreamed and America, the "marvel of nations" banners the skies with the stars and stripes. Marcus Whitman and Lewis and Clarke dreamed long and hard and the bones of oxen and men and women and babies made a bridge over the desert sands and the mountain gorges to the shores of the Sundown Sea, and now the Pullman cars come safely over. Morse and Marconi and Edison dreamed strange wild dreams and concentrated intelligence springs from carbon-crucible and says to earth's boundaries, "Lo; here am I."

Vibration of etheric substance
  Causing light through regions of space,
A girdle of something enfolding
  And binding together the race—
And words without wires transmitted,
  Aerial-winged, spirit-sandalled and shod:
Some call it electricity,
  And others call it God!

A mechanic dreamed, and sprank upon his automobile, and drove it till the axles blazed and the spaces shriveled behind him. Men of high strung airy brains dreamed wondrous dreams, and now the eagle's highway and the open road of men lie parallel.

A musician dreamed a sweet, harmonious dream, and forth from a throat of brass directed by a million tiny fingers of steel, came the entrancing notes that had run riot through the singer's brain.

So let us dream on, men and women, of the day of rest that is already dawning in the heavens. No wonder that Paul said, "How, brethren, are we the Sons of God, but it doth not yet appear what we shall be,"—as such. The morning light of that glad day now purples the mountains of faith and hope with its rays of glory.

And when Man is once fully alive to his own heritage, realizing the wonders and possibilities of his own body, and the power of his soul to control it, and to provide for its needs, he will assert the divine right within him to be a soul in command of its own temple, and the environments of that temple, and will rejoice in the revealed truth of his own divinity that alone can make him free.

The universe is a self-existing, self-winding, self-operating machine. Within its marvelous mechanism dwells every grade of intelligence. From minute molecules to the dynamic thunderbolt, or the microscopic bit of iron that carries a lilliputian atom of oxygen through the blood of prince or pauper, or through the sap of an orange or upas tree, absolute law and order reigns supreme. All substance is a manifestation of motion. All motion is intelligence in action.

The Cosmos, as a whole, must be a being, because it constitutes all intelligence. If there be imperfection, it must be the effect of the infinite word or command.

Man is a product of chemical action. Stellar rays, angles or angels, are the creators of forms. "Let us make man." One lord (planetary) could not make man's body, nor any form of matter. "Us"—the co-operation of planets—makes man.

If a clockmaker can tell how long a clock will run without winding, shall not Being know the days and years of its handiwork? As the maker of a clock oils the machinery in order that it may run with the least friction, and not vainly try to cause a 24-hour clock to run eight days, so shall the coming chemic-astro man supply his body with the dynamic minerals that vitalize and propel red blood through veins and arteries, not to prolong that physical existence, but to attain mental and physical poise until the stellar angles (angels) shall transmute the body, created for soul, into primal float.

Biologists and physiologists have searched long and

patiently for a solution to the mystery of the differentiation of material forms. No ordinary test can detect any difference in the ovum of fish, reptile, bird, beast, or man. Chemical analysis reveals the same mineral salts, carbon, oil, fibrine, albumen, sugar, etc., in the life cell, or ovum, in the blood, tissue, hair, or bone of the multiple and varied expressions of life in material forms.

The Chemistry of Life answers the "Riddle of the Sphinx," and writes above the temple door of investigation, "Let there be light." There is no such things as dead or inert matter. All is life. A crystal is an aggregation of living organisms. The base of all material manifestation is mineral. "Out of the dust,"—ashes or minerals—of earth, physical man is made.

The twelve mineral salts of lime, iron, potash, sodium, silica and magnesium are the foundation stones of every visible form of animal or vegetable. No two forms of the different species of animals have the same combination of this "rock foundation," but all have some of the same minerals. These inorganic salts are the twelve gates of precious stones described in the vision of St. John on the "Isle of Patmos," the pineal gland in the upper brain, the "pinnacle of the temple," the organ of concentration and inspiration.

When the Divine Chemist speaks the atoms of its body—energy—into a certain formula, or combination, a germ or egg-seed, which is a nucleus of the special form to be manifested, commences the process of materialization and persists under the guidance of "God within the shadow, keeping watch above His own." The plexus of intelligent atoms by the law of chemical affinity (a scientific term to express God's creating) attract to the embryo that all pervading something until the "word made flesh dwells amongst us." The building of a body is completed under this Divine Chemistry, according to the plan of the designer.

The constituent parts of man's body are perfect principles, but the principles are not always perfectly adjusted. The planks, bricks, or stones of which a building is to be erected are composed of perfect principles—namely, oxygen, hydrogen, carbon, lime, iron, silica, potassium, magnesia, etc.—but while these principles may be eternally perfect, per se, they may be endlessly diversified in combination.

The stone the builders rejected is symbolized by the stone the builders of the pyramid of Cheops failed to place in position on the top corner—the pyramid being five-cornered, one corner pointing upward, and representing the sense of seeing; so the builders of the science of medicine have failed to place the mineral basis of blood—the inorganic salts—in their place in the human structure or fleshly pyramid.

When these mineral (stone) principles, or elements, are perfectly placed in the chemical formula that composes blood, the animal functions proceed in harmonious operation. When for any reason these cell-salts, stones, are deficient or negative, or dormant, or misplaced, i. e., out of combination, the stone that must become head of the corner has been rejected by the chemistry of life builders.

The human body, or pyramid, is a storage battery, and must be constantly supplied with the proper elements—chemicals—to set up motion or vibration at a rate that will produce what we are pleased to call a live body. A failure to keep this storage battery supplied with the chemical base of blood causes a disturbance in the operation of the chemical action of the blood, the effect of which is called disease. To give names to these effects is the insanity of science.

A lack of the knowledge of the unity or completeness of being, or the perfection of the body or temple of being, was symbolized by the allegory of the temple, or pyramid of Cheops, the capstone rejected—or not yet placed in perfect position. The mineral salts—rock foundation of the human structure—have been rejected by the medical builders for two thousand years or more, but are now, as the earth swings into the air age, Aquarius, the age of Spiritual Man, being recognized as the "Head of the Corner." Thus we see why the beautiful name, Biochemistry, has shown forth from the slowly crystalizing carbon of dead and dying isms and pathies, and now glitters like a diamond in the crown of science. Biochemistry is the "stone the builders rejected."

The fundamental principles of this wonderful science may be outlined in a few words:

Biochemistry, or the Chemistry of Life, uses as remedies the twelve inorganic salts, as found in healthy human blood. These salts are found in all nature—in the food we eat, in the earth, rock, soil, and vegetable, and especially noticeable in mineral springs. They are not taken as medicine, for no medicine, in the common use of the word, is or can be needed. They are taken as food, to supply a deficiency.

But the question naturally arises, why does a deficiency occur if the food we eat contains the mineral salts? The answer is simple: Because the digestion and assimilation sometimes fail to set them free from the organic parts of the food, so that the absorbents can take in a sufficient quantity to keep the blood properly balanced: or some extra demand has been made upon the system—overwork, physically or mentally, atmospheric or electric changes, etc.—which has too rapidly consumed the vitality of the body.

It is then that Biochemistry comes to the rescue. The inorganic vitalizing principles of food having been set free by chemical process, or prepared direct from the mineral base, are give as a remedy, and are taken in by the absorbents at once, not passing through the process of digestion at all, as they are ready for the blood when taken.

There is no such thing as disease, therefore there cannot be any cure, as commonly understood. The symptoms called disease, and named in Latin and Greek, so that the masses are awed and frightened by the very sound of them, are not things or entities—are not something to be combatted, but are simply and only the words, the dispatches, the language Nature employs in calling for that which is lacking.

A shadow cannot be removed by chemicals, neither can disease be removed by poisons. There is nothing

—no-thing—to be removed in either case; but there is a deficiency to be supplied. The shadow may be removed by supplying light to the space covered by the shadow. So symptoms, called disease, disappear or cease to manifest when the food called for is furnished.

The human body is a receptacle for a storage battery, and will always run right while the chemicals are present in proper quantity and combination, as surely as an automobile will run when charged or supplied with the necessary ingredients to vibrate or cause motion.

There can be but one law of chemical operation in vegetable or animal organisms. When man understands and co-operates with that life chemistry, he will have solved the problem of physical existence. When the arteries contain a sufficient quantity of the cell salts, the aerial elements that form the organic portion of blood are drawn into them by chemical affinity or magnetic attraction, and precipitated or concentrated to the consistency that forms the substance known as blood.

The quality of blood depends entirely upon the chemical mineral base. If one or more of the inorganic salts are deficient in quantity, the blood will be deficient in vital or magnetic vibration and cell and tissue-building substance. And so, to supply the organism with the mineral principles that form the positive pole of blood is the natural law of cure. Lymph and lymphatic system is a part of the complex wonderful operation in the process of transmuting the etheric

————51————

substance—aerial elements—into blood, flesh, and bone.

The word, Biochemistry, is formed from bios, the Greek for life and chemistry. Webster defines bio-chemistry as that branch of science which treats of the composition of substances and the changes which they undergo. Therefore, biochemsitry, taken literally, means that branch of science which treats of the com-position of living substances, both animal and vege-table, and of the process of their formation. But usage has given the word a somewhat different signification, and the following is a more accurate definition: That branch of science which treats of the composition of the bodies of animals and vegetables, the processes by which the various fluids and tissues are formed, the nature and cause of the abnormal conditions called disease, and the restoration of health by supplying to the body the deficient cell-salt.

The chemical composition of tissue and the various fluids have long been known, but until Biochemistry was introduced, no practical use had been made of this knowledge in the treatment of the sick. The so-called science of medicine has no claim to the name science. I refer to the old system that treats disease as an entity—a something, or at least caused by a something instead of a deficiency which all must admit to be a lack of something. It is useless for those who adhere to the practice of the drug system to try to defend it. We have the testimony of many of their most noted professors and authors that their "system of practice is responsible for more deaths than war, pestilence, and famine combined."

We realize that modern surgery is an exact science.

Like watch-making or house-building, its purely mechanical. In anatomical exactness, and in instruments
of precision, the advances in surgery during the past
fifty years have been marvelous. While the diagnosis
of disease by surgeons is many times at fault, sometimes fatally so, yet their mechanical operations are
beyond criticism.

Homeopaths builded better than they knew. In preparing their high potencies, they eliminated the poison
contained in such drugs as aconitum and belladonna,
and left only the inorganic cell-salts which supply
deficiences when correctly selected.

Biochemistry is science, not experimentalism. It is
no mystery or miracle, it is natural laws. The food
and drink taken into the stomach, and the air breathed
into the lungs furnish all the materials of which the
body is composed. By the juices of the stomach,
pancreas, and liver, the food is dissolved, and the cell-
salts are taken up by the absorbents and carried to
the lungs, where they unite with the aerial elements
to make blood.

The blood supplies the materials necessary for forming every tissue and fluid in the body, and for carrying
forward every process in the operation or materialization of the human form. An analysis of the blood shows
that it contains organic and inorganic matter. The
organic constituents are sugar, fats, and albuminous
substances. The inorganic constituents are water and
certain minerals, commonly called cell-salts or tissue
builders. Of a living human body, water constitutes
over seven-tenths, the cell-salts about one-twentieth,

organic matter the remainder.

Not until recently were the inorganic cell-salts understood and appreciated. Being little in quantity, they were supposed to be little in importance. But now it is known that the cell-salts are the vital constituents of the body—the workers, the builders,—that water and organic substances are material used by these workmen to carry on the cellular operation in the human organism that underlies and forms the basis of all animal or vegetable tissue. Should a deficiency occur in one or more of these twelve workmen, abnormal conditions arise. These abnormal conditions are known by the general term, disease, and accordingly as they manifest in different ways and in different parts of the body, they have been designated by various names. But these names totally fail to express the real trouble. Every disease which afflicts the human race is due to a lack of one or more of these inorganic workers. Every pain or unpleasant sensation indicates a lack of some constituent of the blood. Does it not naturally follow that the proper method of cure is to supply to the blood that which is lacking?

Deficiences in the cell-salts produce pains, fever, spasms, or some other cry of distress. These so-called symptoms are words, or dispatches, calling for what is needed; and when the call is for the phosphate of potassium to supply nerve cells, shall we give morphine? —"He asked for bread, and ye gave him a stone." When the call is for phosphate of iron, in order that more oxygen may be conducted through the organism, and thereby increase vitality, shall we give alcohol?— "He asked for fish, and ye gave him a serpent."

It will be observed that there is nothing miraculous
about the biochemic procedure—it is simply natural
law. Harmony cannot be obtained when deficiencies
exist by introducing a poison into the system. The
symptoms may be changed to those that manifest differently, but the patient is not cured. Calomel does
not cure; it simply sets up a diarrhoea in place of
constipation. Opium does not cure; it sets up paralysis
of nerve centers in place of neuralgia. Calomel,
aconite, belladonna, salicylic acid, opium, etc. (not re-
ferring to the homoeopathic triburations of these drugs),
are not constituent parts of blood, are not found in
the human organism naturally, and when taken into
the system, set up their own rate of vibration or
action, in place of the condition naturally produced by
a deficiency in the component parts of the organism,
and are worse than the diseases for which they are
given. When a twig is broken from a branch we know
a new one will grow again to the same size if water
is supplied to the soil, and conditions favorable to
its growth are furnished; we do not expect to supply
a new growth by legerdemain, or some short cut—say
by putting an "active poison" about the roots of the
tree, or injecting beneath its bark a nameless lymph
wherein sport the festive bacilli and all-pervading
microbes. We realize the branch must be restored in
a natural manner by the constituent parts of the tree
operating or circulating through the physiology of the
tree, and thus carrying on the process of growth.

Biochemistry has been, and is now being recognized
by the most advanced thinkers the world has known.

Professor Virchow, in his lecture on "Cellular

Patholgy," (Lecture 14) says:

"The cells of the organism are not fed: they feed themselves. The absorption of matter into the interior of the cells is an act of the cells themselves."

Alfred Binet, a noted French scientist, says, in his work, "The Psychic Life of Micro-organism:"

"The micro-organisms do not nourish themselves in-discriminately, nor try to feed blindly upon every substance that chance may throw in their way. The microscopic cellule in some manner knows how to choose and distinguish alimentary substances from particles of sand."

So I am led to believe that the cells are intelligent organisms and can choose their own nourishment. This being the case, how foolish, if not criminal, to place only a poisonous agent within their reach!

As the researches of Binet, the French scientist, show that micro—organisms—infusoria—select their own food from the material at hand, so does the German scientist, the great Virchow, clearly demon-strate that the cells which build the human form divine also select their nourishment from material within reach, and that nothing foreign to their con-stituent parts can be forced upon them—except to produce injury or death. Professor Virchow's re-searches demonstrate the fact that abnormal cells are caused by a lack of the chemical constituents that are required to produce normal cells.

The renowned Dr. Schuessler says: "The inorganic substances in the blood and tissue are sufficient to heal all diseases that are curable at all. The question whether this or that disease is, or is not, dependent on the existence of germs, fungi, or baccili, is of no importance in biochemic treatment. If the remedies are used according to the symptoms, the desired end, that of curing disease, will be gained in the shortest way. Long-standing, chronic diseases, which have been brought about by overdosing or use of poisonous drugs, quinine, mercury, morphine, alcohol, etc., may be cured by minute doses of cell-salts."

Professor Liebig, the world-wide authority in chemistry, says:

"It happens that a tissue in disease reaches such a degree of density, becomes so clogged, that the salt solution of the blood cannot enter to feed and nourish; but if for therapeutic purposes a solution of salt be so triturated and given so diluted that all its molecules are set free, it is presumable that no hindrance will be in the way of these molecules to enter the abnormally condensed part of tissue."

The body is made up of cells. Different kinds of cells build up the different tissues of the body. The difference in the cells is largely due to the different mineral salts that enter into their composition. If we burn the body, or any tissue of it, we obtain the ashes. These are the mineral or inorganic constituents of the body, the salts of iron, lime, magnesium, etc. They are the tissue builders and both the structure and vitality of the body depend upon their proper quantity and distribution in every cell.

Professor Huxley said:

"Those who are conversant with the present state of biology will hardly hesitate to admit that the conception of life of one of the higher animals as the summation of the lives of a cell aggregate, brought into harmonious relation and action by a co-ordinative machinery formed by some of these cells, constitute a permanent acquisition to physiological science. I believe it will, in a short time, become possible to introduce into the human organism a molecular substance that will by the law of chemical affinity find its way to the particular group of cells or nerve plexus that may be in need of it."

"But," you ask, "how does all this consensus of expert authority agree with the germ theory the wise men have been exploiting for so long?"

The true physician, or scientist, says, with Emerson, "I will proclaim what I believe to be true today, though it contradicts what I have advocated all my life."

The true thing alone is orthodox, and no length of time can sanctify error. Not many years ago, the State Board of Health of Louisiana caused cannons to be fired in the streets of New Orleans expecting the concussion to kill the germs of yellow fever. Virchow's research has already completely overthrown the germ or microbe theory of disease.—To be continued.

Germs, or infinitesimal organisms found in disease,

are the product of decaying organic matter—sugar, oil, albumen, etc.—that has left the vital course; and in finding its way to some orifice of the body, it ferments, disintegrates, and thus becomes non-functional. Here we have the cause of a large class of microbes. They are the product of decaying matter caused by a lack of certain cell-salts, which produces a disturbance in the molecular chain of mineral workmen in the body, and thus leaves certain organic matter to be gotten rid of.

It is claimed by the adherents of the germ theory that so-called malarial conditions are caused by germs. Dry air cures ague. Cold weather cures ague. Sodium sulphate—one of the cell-salts of the blood—cures ague. So, then, these must all be Royal Germ Killers! I say no. They supply deficiencies. Ague is caused by an excess of water in the blood, and dry air (cold air is dry air) furnishes an extra amount of oxygen to the blood through the lungs, and eliminates the excess of hydrogenoid gases or water. Sodium sulphate molecules eliminate an excess of water from the system. Each molecule has the chemical force to carry two molecules of water. No one ever has ague whose blood is properly supplied with sodium sulphate, no matter how many germs of malaria may assail him.

We are told by some of the seers of medicine that the biochemic remedies are "harmless" (more than can always be said of their remedies) "and will not hurt a flea"—and they are quite right so far as the flea is concerned. Then what kills the microbe and quickly restores the patient?

The cell-salts do not kill microbes—they supply deficiency that allows organic matter to disintegrate and produce microbes.

The Homeopathic News published the following in an editorial on the germ theory in 1892:

"It is to be hoped that no intelligent homeopath believes in a microbic origin of disease. It may be a matter of interest to the physician to study the bacteriological accompaniments of a given malady—if the malady have any; but the idea that the fullest knowledge of the particular bacillus that may be found in the body of the subject of a given disease is of practical benefit to anybody is a mistake.

"For whether we empirically administer drugs, hoping to cure the disease, or prescribe experimentally for the destruction of a bacillus known to us microscopically, is all one. Give us a specific for cholera, and we care not whether our specific cures by destroying certain bacilli, or by producing blood changes, or in any other way. Where there is no guiding law for the cure of disease, it is all try, try, try, let the cause within the organism be animal, vegetable, or mineral, known or unknown.

"But we do not believe that if bacilli peculiar to certain maladies have been found, they are the cause of the diseased state that they accompany, any more than we believe that the leaves on the tree are the cause of the existence of the tree.

"When a theory of the causation of disease is backed

by names almost universally admitted to be as great as those that endorse the germ theory, intelligent men are willing to investigate it. This we have done most thoroughly; and we believe the theory to be erroneous from top to bottom, and from first to last. We have never found a particle of evidence that bacilli have been discovered—in the sense pretended by their 'discoverers'; and having undoubtedly been 'faked' to a very great extent, beyond doubt intentionally on the part of the chief promulgators of the germ theory, the medical profession cannot be blamed if its members very much doubt whether those gentlemen themselves believe in their own theory, or in their own 'discoveries!' We have learned to know that disease is not an entity, but a condition produced by deficiencies, and that germs are a product of these conditions, and do not cause the conditions."

Those who contend that an effect is a cause cite the fact that a nursing child is liable to contract the same disease the mother may have. The writer of this article was asked by Homeopathic News to explain this important phenomenon in 1893. The following is my answer, which, after so many years, I still present as clear, scientific and logical, and altogether indisputable, because so absolutely true:

"The remark is frequently heard that the baby 'nursed' its sore throat or bad cold from its mother. The statement is not only dogmatic and crude, but in the light of Biochemistry, is unscientific.

"The new pathology claims to be able to scientifically demonstrate the fact that so-called disease is simply a condition, and not an entity, that may be transferred from one to another. Therefore, the expression, 'Caught it from its mother,' cannot be correct."

"But then, the question arises, How shall certain facts be explained? No one will venture to deny that nursing infants are very liable to suffer fom the same symptoms that manifest themselves in their mothers, and when we take issue with the race belief as to the modus operandi by which the condition of the mother appears in the child, it is meet that we should offer our reasons and suggest the true cause of the phenomena.

"In order to make the matter clear, I will offer an illustration: Suppose a child, say five or six years of age, should be fed on a certain kind of grain, known to be deficient in phosphate of lime, and should, as a consequence, suffer from the disease or condition known as rickets, or rachitis, admitted by all schools to be caused by a deficiency of the lime salts of the blood. In such case, no one would maintain that the grain gave the child the rickets, or that it caught it from the grain, but rather that the grain, being deficient in lime, but not in albumen, furnished the blood with a sufficient quantity of organic matter, but not enough mineral or inorganic matter to build up true bone structure.

"Now for the application. Before the mother (or any one else) can have a cold or sore throat, there must be a deficiency in one or more of the inorganic cell-salts or tissue-builders of the blood. Let us suppose the salt that has fallen below the maximum to be kali muriaticum, and, as a consequence, a certain portion of fibrin not having workmen—molecules of kali mur—to use, it was thrown out by the circulation and clogged the parotid gland or tonsils or other glands, or caused irritation to the membrane in nasal passages, or larynx, or bronichial tubes, or pleura, or clogged the air cells of the lungs. In such case, is it not reasonable to suppose the milk would likewise be deficient in the cell-salt, kali mur, and that the child, in accordance with the law laid down above, would also suffer from the result of the deficiency, as did the mother?

"As to germs, or bacilli, or microbes, etc., they swarm throughout all nature. They are Omnipresent Life in operation. They adhere to membranes in unhealthy conditions, but do not effect healthy ones.

"Decaying organic matter produces microbes that exist while the process of decay goes on, feed upon it, and disappear with it, returning to the elements from which they were materialized."

A child may touch a button that will start a complex machine to operating, and yet not understand the science of physics, nor know a thing about the mechanism of the machine.

So it naturally follows that many systems of healing may be the means of starting the workmen in the system that have become dormant into action. Massage, bathing, electricity, magnetic healing, suggestion, absent treatments, concentration, affirmations, prayer, all these and many more that might be mentioned, can and often do start forces that have become dormant because some link in the chemical chain of inorganic molecules has been misplaced or thrown out of gear, but when these chemicals,—for man's body is a chemical formula, remember!—are deficient in the blood, you can no more supply them by any of these modes of operation than you can cure hunger by them. These methods are all good in their time and place to start dormant energies, but none of them will supply deficiencies—that is, satisfy hunger.

Thus, Biochemistry furnishes the key to all cures made by the old or allopathic, the homoeopathic or electric schools, or by medical springs, or healing through the operation of the mind. There are some who heal by thought transference, others must come in contact with the patient. In either case, I hold the process to be orderly, and within the domain of law.

The action of pure, good thoughts, especially directed to restore health, starts a flow of healthy magnetic current which causes assimilation of food in the system, which at once furnishes or sets free the twelve cell-salts and sets them to work—thus cures are made very quickly in many instances. I have been asked many times about the cures made by Jesus of Nazareth. My answer is that He did not violate a single law of nature. He cured by the one law—the Chemistry of Life.

This science is in perfect harmony with the Chemistry of Life operating in each human organism, and cannot antagonize any phase of higher thought. Mind or mental cures, Christian or Divine Science, suggestive therapeutics, or magnetic healing, must all operate according to Divine Law (Life Chemistry) or not at all. The operation of wisdom has many names, but the **chemical process** is one.

"O yes," you say, "it is all very beautiful and wonderful, but after all, can we be sure that it is anything more than a splendid dream?"

To many, it may, indeed, be that, but to many others it is already the truest of all proven facts. And to those who "have not seen, and yet have believed" sufficiently at least, to share in the glory of the dream, I would say, with notes of conviction, and assurance:

Let us dream on, men, women, and babes, of the royal road to health and happiness that is enlightened by the radiance of Biochemic freedom from the drug evil that so long has been a menace to human life and happiness. The darkness shall pass away; poison shall no longer be given to the sick and suffering. The laughing babe shall be a joy to its parents, restored from illness by the principles of life, and rejoicing in health as its guardian angel. The mother shall walk up the pathway of life, beautiful, happy, and contented, rejoicing in her wifehood and motherhood, because no disease lurks within the holy temple of her being. Her husband shall walk by her side in manhood's vigor, with firm step, steady nerves, clear eyes, and balanced mind, no alcohol to fire the blood or scorch and sear the tissue kept swept clean, and sacredly devoted to the dwelling of a soul divine. No poison shall debilitate membranes, destroy the wonderful mechanism of the ear, or cloud the glorious windows of the soul.

Then it shall "follow as the night the day," that quarrels, bickerings, strife, and senseless war shall cease, and in their place shall reason sit enthroned, bathed in the white light of science.

"For behold," cries the New Age, "I come to make all things new."

"THE NEW NAME."

"And I will write upon him the name of my God."
"And I will write upon him my NEW NAME."—
Revelation.

A soul struggling up to the sunlight,
　Up from the mire and clay,
Fighting through wars and jungles,
　And sometimes learning to pray—
And sometimes a king with a scepter,
　And sometimes a slave with a hod—
Some people call it Karma,
　And others call it God.

A beggar ragged and hungry,
　A prince in purple and gold,
A palace gilded and garnished,
　A cottage humble and old—
One's hopes are blighted in blooming,
　One gathers the ripened pod—
Some call it Fate or Destiny,
　And others call it God.

Glimmering waters and breakers,
    Far on the horizon's rim,
White sails and sea gulls glinting
    Away till the sight grows dim,
And shells spirit-painted with glory,
    Where seaweeds beckon and nod—
Some people call it Ocean,
    And others call it God.

———

Cathedrals and domes uplifting,
    Spires pointing up to the sun,
Images, altars and arches,
    Where kneeling and penance are done—
From organs grand anthems are swelling,
    Where the true and faithful plod—
Some call it Supersitition,
    While others call it God.

———

Visions of beauty and splendor,
    Forms of a long-lost race.
Sounds and faces and voices,
    From the fourth dimension of space—
And on through the universe boundless,
    Our thoughts go lightning shod—
Some call it Imagination,
    And others call it God.

———

Acids and alkalis acting,
    Proceeding and acting again,
Operating, transmuting, fomenting,
    In throes and spasms of pain—
Uniting, reacting, creating,
    Like souls "passing under the rod"—
Some people call it Chemistry,
    And others call it God.

Vibration of Etheric Substance,
   Causing light through regions of Space.
A girdle of Something, enfolding
   And binding together the race—
And words without wires transmitted,
   "Ariel"-winged, spirit-sandaled and shod-
Some call it Electricity,
   And others call it God.

———

The touch of angel fingers
   On strings of the human soul.
Anguish and ripples of laughter
   Written across its scroll.
Chords from the holy of holies—
   From sunrise sky to the sod—
Some people call it music,
   And others call it God.

———

Earth redeemed and made glorious,
   Lighted by Heaven within;
Men and angels face to face,
   With never a thought of sin—
Lion and lamb together
   In flowers that sweeten the sod—
Some of us call it Brotherhood,
   And others call it God.

———

And now the sixth sense is opened,
   The seventh embraces the whole,
And, clothed with the Oneness of Love,
   We acknowledge dominion of Soul—
And in all Life's phases and changes,
   And along all the paths to be trod,
We recognize only one power—
   One present, Omnipotent God.

MOONSHINE OR LUNACY?

————

"Is it possible that an insane man may see and express a great truth? Is it necessary to become insane in order that we may cognize the esoteric reality? Do you believe that I am insane? Do you realize that there are many simple problems that will never be solved by so-called 'sane' persons?"

The above questions, and a dozen more along the same line, were hurled at me in rapid succession by the "Moon Explorer," as he persisted in calling himself.

During the summer of 1904, I was traveling salesman for a St. Louis Pharmacy Co. A business engagement called me to Portland, Maine. One evening, I took a trolley ride out to the government fortifications on the bay. I wore my Grand Army button, and was admitted to the army Parade Ground, although it was not Visitors' Day.

The officer, Major Lincoln, was an affable and altogether agreeable host. After dress parade, we strolled through the fortifications and talked on many different subjects. I found that the major was quite enthusiastic on the subject of Astrology and Astronomy, and especially interested, at that particular moment, in everything pertaining to the Moon.

It was the evening of the Full Moon in July—on Moon's Day, too, and curiously enough, in a Lunar hour—and Major Lincoln remarked:

"In a few minutes, the Moon will arise as she has for untold ages, so far as we know, and yet, with all our boasted wisdom, with our telescopes, and spectroscopes, and marvelous instruments of precision for measuring, weighing, and analyzing, we know almost absolutely nothing about the Moon. Why, don't you know." he continued, "that one of our most noted astronomers who enjoys the privilege of looking at the Moon through a forty-inch telescope was recently quoted as saying, 'I know nothing about the Moon, its degree of density, weight, real size—as only one side is ever seen—nor how it came to be where it is, how long it has been there, nor what office it fills in the Solar System!' Some acknowledgment that!—eh?"

The Major leaned over and rested his elbows on one of the mighty guns that lies open-throated towards the in-coming tides ever ready to speak the eloquent language of war, and fixed his eyes on the orb of night, now an "hour high." As I studied his features, I thought,

"What a shame that a man of so finely-balanced head and physique (or any 'image of God' for that matter) should have to devote his life to the brutal, senseless, and altogether unnecessary business of war!"

After a minute or two, Major Lincoln consulted his watch, and smilingly remarked, "We must go outside or the guard will run us in, for it will soon be 9 o'clock—'Taps!'"

As we walked out, I asked the Major if he thought the Moon problem would ever be solved.

"I do not know," he answered gravely, "but we have a very strange specimen of the genus, 'Scientific Hobo rara,' here—commonly defined, 'Tramp-in-ordinary,' who says he knows all about the Moon. He even claims that he has been there, and says that he is the pioneer Moon Explorer. In fact, he declares that there is a good road to the Moon."

I laughed as I answered carelessly, "Why don't you have him locked up? He is evidently 'luny.'"

"Just my idea," replied the Major, though I noticed he had no answering smile for my bantering tone, and rather winced at the attempted pleasantry. After a pause, he added, seriously, "There is a mystery about the fellow I cannot fathom. Insane, of course—there's no question about that, but—well, at any rate, I would like to have you meet him. He lives in that house-tent over there"—pointing to the tent about one hundred yards away—"and as he has made himself very useful to me in many ways, i have been glad to have him remain. He's quite harmless, I assure you. His principal hobby now is to find a person who was born on his birthday, September 7th."

"Well," I remarked, "perhaps he will find in me the fellow he is looking for. My mother seems to rather cling to the idea that I was born on September 7th."

"By Jove!" exclaimed the Major, "is that a fact? How remarkable! Come! You must see him at once!" As "Taps!" were then heard for "Lights out!" the Major added, "The last car leaves for the city at 10, so you will have a full hour to interview 'Moon Explorer'—by the way, he never says the Moon!''

We hurried over to the tent, and found the Explorer of Luna lying on the grass outside the tent, gazing at Moon. The Major said to him,

''This gentleman tells me that he was born September 7th. I will leave him with you, as I must return to the barracks.'' Then, bidding me "Good Night!" after a warm invitation to call again, he walked rapidly away.

Moon Explorer sprang up quickly and gripped both my hands in his, gazing eagerly into my eyes, as one who would search their depths for hidden treasure. Then, with a sigh of relief and gratification, he said:

"I believe you. You look it!—rather tall, slim, light muscles, full of fire and vim and energy, wiry, alert, much like myself—yes, you certainly must have been born on September 7th."

I told him that I must return to Portland on the 10 o'clock car, and that our visit must therefore be brief.

"True," he replied, "and as Virgo people have the faculty of acting quickly—doing it NOW—I will proceed to business—for business it is, my friend, and such as you will certainly be fascinated by. When Mercury, the lord of our lives, lured you to this planet to be, like all of his children, ' a Messenger of the Gods,' he had a mission for you to perform, and for that reason chose the mystic 7th to be your natal day. Do you understand?"

I was plainly mystified, and shook my head with such an air of bewilderment that he hastened to add, "Never mind! If not now, very soon! No son of Mercury can sleep long." He went into the tent-house and returned with a package carefully tied in oil-cloth. "Here," he said, "is a manuscript in which is recorded the most wonderful event the world has ever known, 'THERE IS A ROAD TO MOON.' Maybe you know it, maybe you don't, but it's an actual demonstrable fact that Moon is attached to Earth by an umbilical cord. Earth is the uterus, the Divine Womb, of the Solar System. Earth is the mother of planets; Sun, Sol, or Soul, the father. Moon is a baby planet, not yet fully born, still held by the umbilical cord, while Earth, as a whole, may be called the womb or uterus of—but no more now. You will soon know all. Good-bye!"

I caught the car, and returned to my hotel. I must confess that my experience during the four hours from 6 to 10 P. M. had nearly upset my nerves. I went out to a coffee-house and called for "a pot of coffee with a stick in it," returning to my room at 11 P. M. determined to read that manuscript if I had to remain awake until morning.

I hastily untied the strings about the oil cloth and unrolled twenty sheets of writing paper completely filled with illustrations and writings. The first picture represented the South Pole region of Earth as a vast circular matrix, the size of Moon, 2,000 miles in diameter, and in the center a mighty mountain, reaching into the heavens fifty or sixty miles, growing dimmer and

dimmer and more transparent until it seemed to melt
in air. This mountain was labeled, "The Umbilical
Cord from Mother Earth to Child Moon." The following is a verbatim copy of the strange manuscript:

"On the shore of the Weddle Sea, South Pole, Womb
of Earth, Latitude, 73 Degrees, 20 minutes, South;
Longitude, 146 Degrees, East, I, Nathan Boswell, record
the following facts:

"At the age of 20, I became engaged to be married to
a girl of 17, whose parents resided in Virginia. Her
name was Endolia Fairchilds. Endolia's father was
a cotton merchant, and during the summer of 1884, he
visited New Orleans on business in company with his
wife and Endolia.

"Yellow fever broke out while the Fairchilds were in
the city, and Endolia was stricken with the dread
scourge, and three days thereafter, died. It was about
2 A. M., on August 28th, that Endolia's spirit left its
body. I was at that time a clerk in a wholesale grocery
store in Baltimore. At 12 o'clock that night, I finished
writing a letter to Endolia in which I expressed great
anxiety for her health, I had grave misgivings about
the trip from the time she informed me that she con-
templated taking the journey with her parents. As I
was sealing the letter, I felt that it would be useless
to mail it. There was a letter-drop in the hall, but I
retired, leaving the letter on my writing-table. At
about 4 A. M., I was awakened by a voice calling my
name, "Nat!" (My name is Nathan.) The voice repeated the name several times, until I finally realized
that it was Endolia calling to me.

"I answered, 'Where are you, and what do you want?'"

"The answer came: 'I have passed from earth-life, and shall not see you again until you join me at the South Pole on your journey to Moon: Go to the South Pole, and you will make a great discoverey. I will guide you to the wonderful region—the womb of Earth—and you will then be shown the road to Moon. You will be instructed in the process of transmuting matter from the third dimensional motion to the fourth dimensional rate, and during the time required, you will be able to visit Moon. You will then return and find one born on the same mystic day as yourself who will publish the facts about the great discovery that will revoluntionize the science of the world, after which you will transmute your physical body into a spiritual body, and join me.'

"And now, after a wonderful journey, I am here near the umbilical cord of Moon. Endolia's spirit is with me and guides me on my way to Moon.''

(Two paragraphs omitted here for good reason.)

"Let no one ever dare to penetrate this Holy of Holies until he fully realizes the sacredness of Motherhood. I stand in the holy presence of the Divine Creative Mother Principle and write that which Earth's inhabitants must finally know, but which they will reject and scoff at until the great cataclysm occurs, about the year 1945, that will break the umbilical cord, and set Moon free.

"I am admitted to this sacred region during the year

1881. I was fitted for the ordeal by the teachings of Endolia, who can appear in material garb, and disappear at will. She has attained and understands the .aw cf the Co-Efficiency of Refraction. Those who care to study this alchemical phase of esoteric philosophy will find much help in 'Scientific Romances,' by C. H. Hinton, B. A. My teacher instructed me in the mysteries of birth of planets. All planets are born of the sexual union of Sun and Earth."

(Here I omit several sentences on account of postal laws, although the world ought to know what they disclose.)

"Vibrations of the highly vitalized and spiritualized essence of Sun's rays upon the inner surface of the vast matrix that constitutes the unknown region about the so-called South Pole impregnates the mother-substance concentrated there, and the foetus of a planet is generated. In this realm of God's Creative Compounds, the sweetest perfumes fill the air, a holy calm prevails, and the unregenerated senses taste ambrosia and hear the deep, subtle. heavenly tones of music likened to nothing except the fingers of the Divine Mother touching the keys of energy. For 26,000 years, the baby planet is nourished in the womb of Earth, and then comes that cataclysmal shock that throws the new world 240,000 miles into space, and also tips the Earth at a different angle. The umbilical cord holds until Earth again becomes impregnated with solar energy; then the cord breaks, and Earth rights itself and remains until the travail of another birth. Between the dates of 1940 and 1945, Moon will break away from Mother Earth and take its place as the planet that will govern the constellation, or zodiacal sign, Aries.

"My teacher conducted me to Moon. We ascended the Umbilical Mountain (the navel of Mother Earth) by means of a car constructed of a semi-transparent material that she called Co-Efficient of Refraction. I am scarcely able to define that term. If you ask a dozen different scientists to define Specific Gravity, you may be surprised to learn that few, if any, can give a good definition of the term, although each one of the dozen may really know when to use the words and how to apply them. If I say that Co-Efficient of Refraction means a substance containing the minimum amount of Mars elements to the maximum amount of Venus, Uranus, and Neptune, thus rendering it transparent, the astrologer who reads this will get some idea of its meaning.

"After we had ascended about fifty miles, the substance of the mountain disappeared, and we did not seem to be going up, but simply forward on a level; while my feet seemed to tread on a substance if I stepped out of the car. I could not see anything at all; all seemed like air.

"Endolia explained that while I was changed in the Co-Efficiency of Refraction in regard to muscle and bone tissue, I still had earth-density in relation to brain and nerves, which was necessary so long as I must return and dwell among men for awhile. I lost all idea of the time, as soon as we entered upon the level, transparent road; but my teacher told me we were twelve hours, according to Earth time, making the journey to Moon.

"Moon is inhabited by souls who have passed from

Earth since the birth of Moon. These souls will remain
and be carried to the planetary angle of Aries, there
to develop into Moon beings, as other souls have de-
veloped on Mars, Jupiter, and other planets. Germs
of vegetation are everywhere and the basis of a beautiful world was shown to me by my teacher.. The dark
side of Moon, so-called—the side not seen by Earth-
beings—is a paradise of light and beauty, the Nirvana
of departed earth-souls—that is, those who have departed since the birth of Moon.

"When I asked how Earth would be lighted at night
after Moon departed, she answered, 'Earth will be
lighted at night, until another planet is born, the same
as it now is in the dark of the Moon—lighted by stars
and planets only.'

"Earth remains in perfect equilibrium after the de-
parture of Moon, until the birth of another planet. The
alchemists, seers, sages, and all the spiritually-illumined
ones who have filled their mission on Earth dwell now
on Moon. Their stay there is principally a condition of
Nirvana or rest, yet these spiritual adepts visit their
mother, Earth, at times, and are the true cause behind
all the real spiritual phenomena that manifests on the
Earth-Plane. These teachers are now inspiring all
advanced thinkers—all who write and talk for peace,
brotherhood, and the co-operative commonwealth.

"The mighty pull of young planet Moon during the
ages that it tugs and strains at the invisible umbilical
cord causes it to swing to and fro across the equatorial
line. In ancient times, Moon, or other planets before
our Moon, were known as the 'Serpent,' because their

course was wavering or 'serpentine.' This irregular
motion is due to the resistance of Earth to the pull or
strain of Moon, which causes spasmodic oscilliations.

"The solar system swings around the mighty circle
of the zodiac in 26,400 years; thus remaining in each
of the twelve signs 2,200 years. When Earth enters the
sign Scorpio, which represents the sexual functions of
the Grand Man of Heaven, she gives birth to a new
planet. Moon makes the eighth planet. There will be
four more, thus making twelve—one for each of the
twelve signs of the Zodiac.

"As I just said, the Solar System remains 2,200 years
in one sign. It entered Aquarius in 1900, and must
pass through Capricorn and Sagittarius before reaching
the celestial Scorpio—on the regenerative plane, Scorpio
becomes the White Eagle—which will require about
6,600 years of Earth-time; and then another child-planet
will be born. This will be the Christ-Child among
planets—the regenerative child of that fluidic, etheric,
electro-magnetic substance which is to be the redeemer
—the saving force—the life-preserving elixir—the
transforming vibratory influence—of the universe.

"Earthquakes are Earth-spasms, vibrations, or
orgasms, caused by the descent of the Sun's magnetic
fluid, which enters Earth at the South-Pole matrix.
From now on, until Moon breaks away, these magnetic
shocks will occur with increased frequency and violence.
Sensual-minded people will be taken out of material
expression in great numbers, but the 'pure in heart'
will survive.

"The climax of Earth-throes will be reached during the year 1916, and those who survive the ordeal will live to see the beginning of the millennial reign of the Aquarian Age—the age of men and women.

"Having been taught the art of transmutation, I shall enter into the new rate of motion, the fourth dimension, and dwell on Moon until that Divine Child goes to its place in the cosmic cycle."

Here the manuscript ended.

Late in December of 1904, I visited Portland again, and called at the military barracks to see Major Lincoln, and ask if Moon Explorer was still there. The Major informed me that the tramp had disappeared on September 7th—the night of the Full Moon—and that no trace of him had yet been found.

I often ask myself whether the manuscript was written by an insane man, or by one with "Method in his madness." Who answers?

————

WAR.

War is the sum of all villainies.

War is the mother of hate, the father of lies, the sister of the great Whore, the brother of the devil.

War makes a charnel house of the world, fills the land with mourning and gibbering; its senseless jargon impedes the onward march of man.

Instead of the occupancy and use of land under peace and co-operation we have the ownership of land made legal by conquest of hellish war—thus the absentee land owner and the tenant slave.

A battleship that costs from $10,000,000 to $15,000,000 lasts from three to five years. Efficiency then 50 per cent; consequently the ship goes to the junk pile.

Requires the wages of three workers at $600 per year to support one soldier.

It costs the nation $400 every time a cannon is discharged.

Nothing is gained by war. All progress is the result of peace and co-operation between people and nations.

The best physical specimens of manhood compose armies, are killed, and thus the race deteriorates physically.

Those who survive have been brutalized by the unspeakable crime of war; thus morality deteriorates.

In order to sell steel, gunpowder and implements of murder, capitalists subsidize newspapers, magazines and schools and churches and thus glorify war, by appealing to patriotism, clothing children in soldier uniform, and teaching them to sing "America," and the "Star Spangled Banner."

The capitalist first appeals to love of country, law and order, then hides his unspeakable villainies under the folds of the Stars and Stripes.

War spells bankruptcy.

Peace spells prosperity.

"War is hell."

THE ANGEL OF PEACE.

I come from the cosmic center
   God's region of light and peace.
I come with the manifesto:
   "Let wars and their rumors cease."
Cease your babble and wrangle
   And muzzle your dogs of war
And brotherhoods creed plain worded
   Shall rise like the morning star.

Let the bugles all sing truce
   Across the blood drenched field
Let all the people join the song
   "Sweet peace shall be our shield"
Let all join in the march to the highlands
   That rise o'er the gloom of night
The purpling peaks of freedom
   That gleam in the morning light.

Come all and join the procession
   With songs of peace for the soul
And God and the angels will help you
   To reach the long-sought goal.
Farewell! I return to my center
   I have given my message of peace
And I pray to the Father in Heaven
   That wars forever shall cease.

WIRELESS MESSAGES CAUGHT BY DR. GEORGE W. CAREY.

————

"Say, Pa, what is the difference between war and preparedness?" There is no difference Johnny, except in the spelling. Now run out and don't ask any more foolish questions.

————

A monkey may be trained to imitate a man. But there are many men who imitate a monkey perfectly without any training whatever. Peg one for Mr. Darwin.

————

Man can measure the distance to the Sun, count the rings of Saturn, the moons of Jupiter and survey the canals on Mars, but he knows no more about the process of digestion, the composition of bile nor the growth of his hair, or how his blood is formed, than a politician knows about the science of government.

————

Man talks of kindness to animals, but he eats beefsteak, mutton chops, veal cutlets and fried chicken daily.

————

Women often feel very sorry for dogs and cats, feed them, clothe them, bathe them, put ten dollar collars on them, take them out in automobiles—while there are hungry children in the next block.

————

Earth is one of the heavenly planets, one of the bunch "up there" not "down here."

A man often speaks about the ignorant foreigner who speaks three languages correctly, while the critic cannot speak his own language as well as a parrot.

———

Yes, Matilda, I think you should have a chaperon provided your chaperon has a chaperon.

———

A man will often talk of microbes in drinking water while trying to get his living from the wet end of a cigarette that smells to heaven and causes angels to hold their noses.

———

The little anarchists, poor men, and the big anarchists, senators, cabinet officers, insurance managers, oil kings, trust magnates, et al., are so numerous that they make the law-abiding middle class look like 15 cents.

———

The universal revolt against authority and so-called laws by rich and poor alike must have a scientific cause. The solar system is now entering Aquarius and the age of reason has commenced.

———

Edison did not obtain the knowledge that enabled him to invent the telephone from books. It was not in books. Edison as a material entity did not invent the telephone. Infinite wisdom, operating through the organism named Edison brought forth into operation the telephone. Universal life or intelligence is not a "prentice hand" that needed practice to evolve the telephone.

The Eternal Cause knew all it knows or ever will know a billion aeons ago and forever.

————

The physical organism of man is an instrument on which Life plays or works, and Life always forms the instrument it needs for the moment, expresses its wish, speaks its word, then "throws the reed away."

SOULS.

————

Souls are thoughts of God.

God is eternal, self-existing.

Souls being God's thoughts are eternal, self-existing. Souls have always been souls, for God has always been God.

God has not evolved. God's desire to manifest, or operate, is shown forth in manifestation or operation of souls.

To call this procedure evolution or progression is meaningless and foolish; to call it operation or manifestation is wisdom.

THE OCCULT MEANING OF SLANG PHRASES.

"Whatever satisfies souls is true."—Walt Whitman.

Great truths are always sensed and crudely expressed first by the common people.

The truth of Campbell's statement, "Coming events cast their shadows before," is nowhere more freely exemplified than in the slang phrases used by nearly all classes, but we find that a large per cent of slang originates with those known politically as "the common people."

Truth has a way of clothing itself in homely attire and thus masquerading before the multitude in order that the cells of the human brain (a mirror in which nature is reflected—invisible principle made visible to mind) may become adjusted to the new concept or phase of infinite operation wrongly named evolution.

Why should one ever say "No matter?"

On its face there seems to be no relevancy whatever, between the phrase and the idea seeking expression.

But chemistry, the "court of last resort," proves that socalled matter is not matter after all, but simply a manifestation or precipitation of energy, force, or aerial elements.

Huxly said at a session of the International Medical

Congress in London, "matter in its last analysis evades me." Herbert Spencer said: "I now believe that there is one universal energy from which all things proceed."

If the appearance, or substance we call "matter" proceeds from energy it must be energy (life or spirit) in the concrete, just as ice is vapor or water crystallized, or water is oxygen and hydrogen in a combination that forms a substance visible and tangible to the physical senses.

The spectroscope, the X-ray, and chemical analysis have quite demonstrated that so-called matter is "no matter" and yet not an illusion or no thing. Matter is spirit or energy in manifestation, and is therefore real.

"Catch on" is a popular slang phrase, but it was borrowed from the cultured Emerson, who said, "Hitch your wagon to a star." There is no difference between "hitch on" and "catch on." Both expressions embody the advice to "aspire" and "be awake."

Edison says he believes there is a universal, though very subtile vibration forever in action, of some unknown substance, ether, or essence, and when we "catch on" to it, the wonders we may perform will transcend the wildest dream of seer, poet or philosopher.

Edison believes that machines may be so nicely adjusted that they will respond in key or tone to this "Divine Strain"—wisdom's pulsing dynamo—and thus be set in motion by the "Universal Energy."

It has recently been demonstrated that so-called electricity is not a fluid or substance of any kind or quality that can pass along a wire, or "go" anywhere, but that it is simply an effect or jar—a vibration.

But for several years before this remarkable fact was established, the boys on the street were saying, "wouldn't that jar you?"

Why did they coin the significant phrase?

Was it because the spirit that breathes into man the breath of life uttered the prophecy of coming events through human phonographs? Do we not really talk out what has been talked into us?

"Nothing doing" is a symbol of Christian Science belief—the unreality of sin, sickness, evil, death and even matter. Some critics of Christian Science contend that the term Christian Science itself clearly accentuates the meaning of "nothing doing," for the simple reason that there can really be no qualifying adjective prefixed to the word "Science." Therefore, when we say "Christian Science," we say "Nothing doing."

"Nobody at Home" is the story of the Prodigal Son in three words. In material concept, the soul or Ego within man's body does not realize that it is spirit now, residing in a house or temple of flesh, and so like the Prodigal Son it wanders about looking for happiness everywhere under the sun except within its own consciousness. Hence the phrase, "Nobody at home" is applicable to all who look for happiness in the spectacular or outward appearances.

The chemists all tell us that we "live, move and have our being" in a highly attenuated element and that all forms of vegetable, animal, or mineral life are but rates of motion of this substance.

But the slang phrase "we are in it" and that terse observation "up against the real thing" have been common expressions for several years.

Of course we are both in and up against this stuff whatever name we select for it and it presses upon us something like fourteen pounds to the square inch of bodily surface.

It is assuredly the "real" thing because there is nothing else for us to be "in" or "against."

Few people these days believe that death ends all, or that the fleshly body is more than a vehicle or diving bell, as it were, for spiritual man's convenience while operating upon the plane of consciousness as one of the attributes of the unnamable Necessity.

Yet we can hardly think that the fellow who says "I won't do a think to him" in any manner realizes that he can't do a thing to the real "him"—the spiritual ego.

Emerson forcibly expressed the Hindu philosophy of this great truth in his poem on Brahm, thus.

"If the red slayer thinks he slays,
Or the slain thinks he is slain,

They little know the subtle ways
I come and pass and go again."

Life—all life—is eternal. It cannot be destroyed. Literally you "can't do a thing to it."

We used, all of us, to say: "We won't do a thing to those Spainards when we get to Cuba." And we did not. Every Spainard that ever lived, still lives, or else immortality is an "iridescent dream."

All is divine. If death, disease, war and disaster are true, they are divine—part of the scheme of things.

Flesh bodies change their rate of motion, drop away and release spirit and are resolved back again into their original elements, but these elements are indestructible.

They are the cells or molecular dynamos of the body of the universe. These atoms are Omnipresent Life in operation. We "can't do a thing" but accept it.

"Come down from the perch" is literally obeyed by the daring aeronaut with parachute and figuratively obeyed by ward politicians, mayors, city councils, legislators, senators, bankers, beef trust and railroad and oil trust promoters, et al., "caught with the goods."

"It is up to you," in an esoteric sense, simply means that you must work out your own salvation without the assistance of crucified Redeemers or saints.

"All right," spoken daily by people of all beliefs—

even by those who think that everything is wrong—is the basis of mental science emphasized by Pope in "whatever is, is right."

The Universe and all it contains is either governed by law or all is chance. It is unthinkable that law is not dominant in all operations or procedures. When we say "all right," we express a truism although we may not personally believe it.

"You are not the only pebble on the beach" is a statement prophetic. It foretells the coming consciousness of unity, as well as an awakening spirit of altruism and brotherhood.

It is a loud protest against selfishness, and caste, or class distinction.

The "whole hog or none" means the One Life, One Cause, or else there is no life and no cause.

We may not use hog flesh for food and yet see that the hog is an expression of the same energy that we see expressed in all the varying forms and so we "go the whole hog."

"Knock the stuffing out of it," typifies the John the Baptist, the iconoclast, the idol-breaker.

It stands for the annihilation of the false idea of the importance of possessions, or as my Saint Whitman says, "the mania of owning things." The cartoons of the present day Trusts are pictures of stuffed men, and

everywhere the people are taking a whack at them trying to "knock the stuffing out of them."

"A chip off the old block" again emphasizes the
Oneness of Substance. We are slices or chips from the
Universal block. "Out of sight," or "way up in G,"
refers to the real or spiritual man, a higher note
(vibration) than the material expression.

"The whole show," or "he or she is the whole show,"
is literally the truth, for man is an epitome of the
macrocosm, and all concept is possible for his understanding.

"Cut it out" is a direct command to cut out of your
life all that retards your harmonious operations.

Cut out the belief in evil as a principle of being, also
the false idea of imperfections. Cut out excuses, complaints, and regrets.

"Up to date" is a phrase often used and indicates an
awakening to the saving truth that there is no passing
time, but instead, the ever present eternal NOW, and
that all operation is up-to-date, or now.

"Get a move on you" is the best slang phrase ever
expressed upon the brain cells of man. It is a strong
suggestion to get out of the rut of a line of thought
that has served its time and is of no further use in
the procedure of wisdom.

Those who think only of self should move up into

the realm of altruism and read Edward Bellamy's "Equality."

Those who believe in evil should move to the last letter and spell the word backward thus: live. Those who live in the swamps of a belief in disease and microbes and devils, big or little, obsession and contagion (being always ready to catch something) should move to the mountain top of belief in Omnipresent Life and there chant the ninety-first psalm. That blessed anthem will fill them with such courage that they will not even fear the kissing microbe nor any of the host of Latin named bugs that doctors tag with labels and

then let loose on the frightened people. The microbe theory of disease is the insanity of pseudo-science, and the people have begun to awake to a realization of the fact.

"Take him down a peg" is well illustrated in the ancient allegory of the Prodigal Son who was over-anxious about his portion of his father's goods. It takes one down a peg when they cognize the great truth that each one has his portion always.

Infinite intelligence would be unjust to withhold one's rightful portion for an instant.

The great DYNAMIS knows its business and never fails in its "perfect returns."

"He is a crank" is simply a truism. A crank is a lever that moves machinery. A human crank is a fellow that moves society—the world.

"Served him just right" was a popular slang during the earlier days of the theosophical movement.

Theosophists look upon the events of one's life here and their daily activities as the result of their former lives and that whatever experience they are called upon to pass through is simply the working out of their karma—be it good or bad, and therefore they are always served right. Those who take a broader view contend that all souls are attributes of the One Soul, and that rewards or punishments are impossible. To "serve" means to wait upon, to assist, to benefit, and the One

Life is always serving or assisting its attributes right. We are all kings and queens and the great Energy is our royal servant, breathing into us life, pulsing our hearts and playing divine harmonies upon the wondrous cells of our brains.

"He has the grit" or "the sand"—or lacks it—has a chemical basis. The base of human bodies as well as all materialization is mineral (sand or grit).

A lack of cell-salts in blood and brain causes weakness and inaction, hence the phrase "lacks grit" is literally true.

Let us not despise slang—even though we do not use it—but rather let us endeavor to comprehend the mighty truth that the wisdom that expressed the words or symbols called "slang" through the organisms of plain and ofttimes illiterate persons is the same wisdom that placed Orion with his clustering lamps in the southern sky; stationed the sentinel Arcturus with his bended bow above the northern pole; holds the heavens in balance with Alcyone and the circling stars of the Pleiades; sends the comet—its swift electric messenger —to creation's outer circle as watchman or messenger with the key to the holy of holies; bearing upon its flaming front a spiritual headlight that casts its beams across measureless wastes of star dust that binds in one, the universe; "whose body nature is, and God the soul."

We are not deceived by the costumes worn by actors upon the drama stage, then let us not be deceived by the disguises in which infinite Wisdom appears upon the stage of material experience.

FREEDOM.

The rain that falls in the heart of man,
  Flows out through the eyes in tears;
And God's decrees in the soul of man,
  Are wrought in the cycle of years.

Mortal thought in the heart of man,
  Is flotsam on life's sea
The divine urge in the soul of man
  Is the word that sets him free.

PARADOXES OF CIVILIZATION.

A man may work faithfully for many weary years as farmer, chopper, carpenter, or in any and every line of necessary labor for the benefit of his fellowman, and as he grows older and less competent to produce a given amount of food or other commodities, his wages are reduced in diverse ratio to his needs; and if by chance, through ill health, accident or other misfortune, he fails to accumulate a competency for old age, he becomes a pauper and goes to the poorhouse. But the man who enlists in the army, puts on military uniform and goes forth to murder men whom he never saw, until he meets them on the battle field, is rewarded with a pension that is increased as he grows older. Thus it comes to pass that the toiler who works to save life and property goes to the almshouse in his old age, while he who devotes his energies to the destruction of life and property is rewarded by the government and guaranteed a living in his declining years. This is the crowning paradox of civilization's monstrous list.

The tyranny of the dead has long been the skeleton at every feast, the "Dweller on the Threshold" of human thought, and the supreme tyrant of the world. This spectre of Eld chatters a jargon of "Precedent" and "Authority," and forever pulls backward at the hands on the dial of Now.

If you have a case in court, its merits will be decided by the rulings of a judge who lived in colonial times, when they burned women for being clairvoyant or intuitive. If you paint a picture, the judges compare it with some old dried paint on a torn and tattered canvas, painted by some one who died before the pyramids were built, or the walls of Karnack were reared above the ancient Nile. And unless it bears some resemblance to the old wreck of paint and canvas, you are voted an amateur, and advised to go to Rome or Venice or Florence and study the old masters.

You may be able to call from out the hidden corridors of the violin or piano vibrations that attract the gods to come your way and honor you, that start every nymph hustling for her dancing costume; but if some professor, with a name twisted and knotty as his brain, does not hear a plagiarism of Beethoven, or Haydn, or Paginini, or Mozart, or some other fellow, ages agone turned to dust, you might as well go to plowing.

If you suggest a live, warm thought on political economy, or tariff, or financial reform, or any line whatsoever, you are met with the rebuff of some learned prig who quotes Jefferson or Adams or Clay or Hamilton or Douglass or Seward or Lincoln, and solemnly reminds you of what these good and wise men—in their day, but long dead—would do if they were here; and for fear you might deviate an inch or so from their standard, you are advised to go slow and wait.

In you dare to think out, in the here and now, a theory of the universe, of the at least seeming intelligence that moves and adjusts matter in orderly sequence, that manifests that which is manifested, and man in his relation to this power, or energy, you are assailed by myriads of angry men and women—backs to the day, facing the cemeteries of the past—and told what Jesus said, or would say or do if he were here, or what Paul,

or John, or James, or Peter, would do, say, or think
about it. And if your theory should be at all sensible,
sane, practical, something you want Now, and that
everybody wants Now, if they could think, you are told
that it is contrary to the opinions and advice of those
dead men, and if you value your soul's salvation, you
must abandon such wicked thoughts.

O that man had no soul to save Then, indeed, he
might act sanely and rationally, and naturally, and no
longer be ruled by the dead!

If you find something in the here and now, about
physiology and materia medica, that bears the scent of
the morning dew, or reflects the light of the noonday
sun, the musty, ill-smelling medical board straightway
wants to know if it is in Dalton's Physiology, or the
prescriptions of Hiprocates, and if you have a diploma
written in Latin.

Let us close the books. Push them back into the
dark corners. Break down the walls of the prison house.
Tear away the roof. Spill the bottled blood of imaginary
redeemers. Burn the musty, moldy parchment containing hieroglyphics of mummied saints, and issue the
Declaration of Independence from the tyranny of the
dead, and all the devils of the past and present.

Let the winds of unshackled thought sweep away
the unpleasant odor of dead gods and decaying Pharaohs. Let us stand in the unwalled and roofless temple of the Kingdom of the Now, lighted by myriad suns,
and bejeweled with countless constellations. Search no

more for the miraculous—the greatest of all miracles is
yourself. I know of nothing but miracles. The greatest
of all times is now. The greatest of all places is here.

This is an age of keen investigation, of truth-finding,
and idol-breaking. He who is afraid to investigate for
fear some cherished idol will be broken is not a true
scientist, and not true to himself.
No length of time ever sanctified anything, and the
truth alone sets free. But how shall we explain the
seeming contradictions that confront us at every turn?

The inconsistencies and paradoxes in the thoughts
and actions of man can be explained only on the
hypothesis that one power, principle or cause does all
and is all, and that so-called paradoxes are but steps
in the operation of wisdom, moving in orderly procedure to the completion of certain phases of expression.

In chemistry, acids and alkalis are paradoxical; being
opposite, the cause chemicalization, or fomentation,
which seems to be confusion. In ancient alchemical
writings, this phrase when applied to human life was
called Babylon, which, when traced to its root, we find
means confusion.

The world's civilization, since recorded history began,
has been one chain of paradoxes. The scales of competition forever tipping cause the phenomena. The pro-
ducers of food starve because they cannot buy the food
they produce. The makers of clothing are in rags
because they can't pay, in the coin of the realm, for
the clothing they make. Prices are too high for the

consumer, or too low to please the producer. If workers demand the full product of their labor, they are denounced as thugs and anarchists by those who do not produce anything. In competitive thought there appears to be many inconsistencies.

Man lays his sceptre on the stars, analyzes their substance, and then dies from the effect of acid in his blood, because he does not know what to eat. He foretells the return of a comet to an hour, but cannot tell if he himself will have la grippe next week. He can tell you the hour in the day one hundred years hence that there will be high tide at Bombay, or along the coast of Norway, but he doesn't know the cause of smallpox, and foolishly thinks the decaying organic matter or pus from a sick calf injected into the blood may somehow prevent it.

He can clothe himself in armor and dive to the ocean's floor, or travel three thousand leagues under the sea in a submarine boat, and then be killed by a street car or automobile in broad daylight on the level road. He knows how to keep the chemicals properly balanced in the storage battery of his automobile, but puts alcohol, morphine and tobacco in his own body and wrecks it.

He can tell all about the moons of Jupiter, the rings of Saturn, the transit of Venus, the canals of Mars, and can talk with the man in the moon, but he knows no more about the real composition of his own blood or nerve fluid or the mysteries of digestion or assimilation, or the chemical formation of bile, than a politician knows of the true science of government.

He can vibrate the air at Boston at a rate that will record the same dots and dashes on a receiver at Liverpool, but cannot receive and correctly translate a dispatch from his solar plexus to his brain.

Why is man forever a paradox? Why does he always want to level down a hill or fill up a hollow? Get married, if single, or get a divorce, if married? Why does he want cold weather when it is warm, and warm weather when it is cold? Why does he lock a man up in jail for begging for food, and then give him three meals a day?

Man declares that he is mortised and based in the statement, "Thou shalt not kill!" and attuned to the music of "Peace on earth, good will to men," and yet the iron-clads do not rust, nor are the battle-flags furled. He loads his musket with the Sermon on the Mount of Olives—emblems of peace—and his cannons with the Laws of Moses, and bombards alike the Dutch farmer in South Africa and the brown men on the Thousand Isles of the Filipinos. He prays for the time to come quickly when "Swords shall be beaten into plowshares, and spears into pruning hooks," but he keeps the sea covered with warships, shakes the solid earth with the tread of soldiers, while the smoke from his arsenals and manufactories of implements of war and murder darken the noonday sun.

Man mutilates his fellow men and then establishes a Red Cross Society and hospitals to care for him and bind his wounds. He invents ways and means to destroy the bodies of men, and if by accident one is not killed outright in battle, surgeons and nurse are called to save his precious life. Every attention is given the wounded prisoner; watchful care, the best food, hygienic conditions and beautiful flowers, all aiding his recovery. And editors write editorials on "Human Warfare," while the masses declare that "Ours is a Christian nation," and the gods stand amazed at the paradox.

Man condemns cruelty to animals, but the slaughter house disgraces civilization, and man expects beefsteak for breakfast. He preaches humanitarianism, but the sweatshops still remain a bloody blotch on the face of humanity. He preaches kindness and gentleness to children, but dresses them in military toggery—gives them tin swords, toy pistols and cannons, drills them in the manly art of self-defense, and tells them to be "strenuous," all under the auspices and sanction of the churches whose walls resound with songs and sermons of "Peace on earth."

Patricts, real statesmen, humanitarians, seers, prophets, the far-seeing, self-sacrificing lovers of humanity, are derided, abused, persecuted, imprisoned, tortured, crucified, and then monuments are erected with cold chiseled marble to mark their burial place; and the poet and historian vie in singing their praises, while their features are preserved on innumerable canvasses, and their sightless eyes stare out from bronze and plaster of paris in every library, or stand sullen and silent in a niche in the Hall of Fame.

Men and women teach the everlasting truth that we are all children of one common mother and father—the eternal Positive-Negative Energy from which all things proceed—and therefore members of one family—brothers and sisters in truth—but they insist upon an introduction before speaking to each other as they pass. Sons of God, and yet they must not greet each other without an introduction! O the pity of it! O the shame! Man asserts that God is love, and then writes in a book, "the fear of God is the beginning of wisdom."

Love is altogether lovely and no one can fear it. Some people are so afraid that they will go to hell when they die that they live in hell all the time on earth. Some are so afraid of smallpox that they poison themselves with vaccine pus, which is more deadly than smallpox.

Socialism means Society, industrial and financial, and organized for the benefit of all equally, where each person receives the full product of his labor, through collective ownership of the tools of production and the means of transportation, where there are no middlemen, no judges to render void the will of the people by the Moloch, "Unconstitutional" — in short, Socialism means the complete organization of society for the public good. Anarchy means no organization of any kind for any purpose whatsoever. Anarchy means no law of a majority or a minority. Anarchy teaches the free and unrestricted liberty of the individual. Frederick Neitzsche, the chief anarchist of modern times, with the possible exception of our Napoleons of finance, says: "Of all men I hate the Socialist the most because he tries to lift the dull ignorant mass of human beings up to a higher plane. My contention is that the individual that realizes that there is a higher plane should strive to reach it unencumbered with the dead weight of ignorance."

Thus is the line sharply drawn between Socialism and Anarchy. But that portion of people and press that derive their income by serving the great business interests repeatedly state that Socialism and Anarchy are one and the same.

This is evidently a paradox with a purpose.

A woman has been known to ride wild horses, shoot deer, panthers and bears, drive horses hitched to a stage coach, pilot a steamboat on the Mississippi River, and then faint dead away when a mouse ran across the floor.

Women are peaceable and kind-hearted, but they do so adore soldiers and warships. They detest tobacco and liquor, but marry men who use both. A woman will express pity and sorrow for the poor and needy, and then put a ten dollar collar on a fat, pudgy dog, and let it lead her along the street, while five orphan children are ragged and hungry on her block. Women love birds—especially on toast; they love the beautiful plumage of birds—especially on their hats.

Man declares the laws enacted by legislatures and congress are sacred. He then violates these laws, carries his case to the court of last resort, and gets the sacred laws repealed. Man declares majority should rule, but bitterly opposes the majority when contrary to his opinion.

Many persons speak of "the ignorant foreigner"—a man who probably speaks three languages correctly, while his critics can't speak their own language as well as a parrot.

The automobile driver may scorch his wagon along the street at a forty-mile clip, if he will toot a horn to warn pedestrians to flee from the wrath coming, but the man on foot is locked up in jail if he runs amuck in the street, shouting, "Get out of my way!" Men say that God is everywhere, and that the devil is everywhere, too, and then proves mathematically that two objects cannot occupy the same space at the same time.

The Christian professes to believe that after the change called the death of the body, his soul will be wafted to a place called Heaven—a place of beauty and eternal peace, where he will have a mansion of gold. windows of precious stones, fronting the pure waters of the River of Life, that flows from the Throne of God: but let that same Christian have a pain in his stomach, and he sends a hurry call to the nearest physician and begs him to use all his skill to keep him here in this vale of tears—here among the "beggarly elements of the world," where he may remain a "worm of the dust" a little while longer.

Mental Scientists affirm health and opulence, and then fail in business and change climate to cure nervous prostration.

Christian Scientists make the very truthful statement

that "God being omnipresent, fills all space, and is all there is or can be"; and then charge three dollars to treat you for "mortal mind thought" and to protect you from "malignant magnetism.

Spiritualists say that the orthodox belief in a personal devil, one big fellow with hoofs and horns, is quite absurd and amusing, and then these reformers will declare that most sickness is caused by evil spirits, and then will offer to cure obsession for five dollars per cure.

A highwayman murders a man for his money, but refuses to eat the dead man's lunch of meat because he must keep the Lenten days.

Physicians experiment with poison, and find that a certain drug will cause disease in the human body, when taken internally; and when called to prescribe for the sick, they administer the drug that causes disease, believing that two diseases are better than one.

The average man declares that woman is far superior to man in perception, intuition, and judgment in regard to social life and the welfare of the family, but he bitterly opposes the franchise for women. Man is not willing that mothers should have a vote in making laws to govern their own sons and daughters. Man seems willing to give to women everything under the sun that they don't need, from chewing gum to china vases, and refuses to give them the thing they need most—the ballot.

Our wives, mothers and sisters may perform all sorts

of labor, study all the arts and sciences, own property and pay taxes, and be amenable to man-made laws; yea, a woman may go down into the dark valley, where God's creative compounds materialize in human form, and kiss the white lips of Pain before she holds a babe to her breast, but she must not have a voice in laws to govern that child. Whatever is unwomanly is also unmanly.

The cry of "hard times" is always heard. People dole out nickels or pennies grudgingly for charitable purposes, or civic improvements, or good roads; but a prize fighter receives a hundred thousand dollars for hitting a fellow on the jaw, men pay five dollars for a bottle of champagne, and two dollars for a porterhouse steak; and a woman will spend forty dollars for a hat that has no more correspondence to the contour of the human body than politics has to honest government, or the co-operative commonwealth.

Men complain of unjust tariffs and taxes, call upon Heaven to witness the iniquity and dishonesty, graft, thievery and fraud of courts and law-makers, and then go meekly to the polls and vote for the same fellows over again.

Tired men and women will squeeze into crowded cars, and step on each other's toes while holding straps; but if you mention municipal or national ownership of railroads as a remedy, they say: "O I do not bother about politics. Which team won the football game?"

Dogs are allowed to roam at will over lawns and amongst the flowers, while little boys and girls stand on the walk and read a sign board, with this strange device, "Keep off the grass!"

Man must be quiet and orderly, must not talk, or laugh in a manner that will disturb the peace of his neighbor; but dogs may bay at the moon and planets, the comet, the dog-star, the Pleaides, or any old thing; and cats may curse and swear, and rip the boards off the woodshed in an unearthly noise contest, and the poor wretch who dares to protest is called "a cruel, bad man!"

If you refuse to cast a ballot on election day, you are denounced by the "fearless press" as an undesirable citizen, but when you do vote, you must take a beating by an election ward thug, have your vote challenged by a "heeler," and then, if you vote against the push, have your vote thrown out as "irregular."

A citizen of the United States reads about the Alps, buys an alpenstock and a ticket for Europe, spends three years abroad, and incidentally spends sixteen thousand dollars. But when the Swiss peasant asks the U. S. citizen about Yosemite, or Shoshone, or Niagara, he is oftentimes amazed to learn that the American tourist has never worshiped at the feet of El Capitan, that he never thrilled with awe as he looked at the descent of Snake River into the awful gorge at Shoshone, nor never bathed in the rainbow mists above tumbling Niagara.

Think of a man going to Europe to see the sights, who has never looked down into the riven earth, where the Colorado canyon reveals Nature's carvings and colors, nor passed through the Enchanted Gateway of the Cascade Mountains, where Jupiter Olympus hurled thunderbolts in the ancient days, and dug a canal between the snow-capped mountains, Adams and Hood, and let the inland lakes flow to the Sunset Sea!

"See Columbia's scenes, then road no more; naught else remains on earth to cultured eyes." Columbia, the "river of the west." The Nile might come from its cloudy heights and pour the water of Egypt into this mighty stream, and it would cause no ripple upon its broad expanse, nor would it increase the speed in its stately march to the sea.

The firs of Oregon and Washington and the redwoods of California equal the Cedars of Lebanon; and the pillars of salt on the shores of Palestine's Dead Sea is outdone by the dead sea on Utah's plains. Truly, the man is a paradox who explores every country on the globe, except his own.

A literal interpretation of the mythological characters, astronomical allegories and alchemical symbols of the Bible has caused earth to run red with bloody wars, and has arraigned neighbor against neighbor in petty quarrels, envy, criticism and hatred.

The belief, based upon literal reading of ofttimes mistranslated texts, that the blood of a man, however good he may have been, could by virtue of an ignominious death save unborn souls from the result of their own ignorance, has made idolators of a large portion of the human race.

It seems incredible that men and nations should have gone to war about God, for the Bible, which is the warrant for all religious wars, says "God is love.".

Yet such has been the case, and such still is the case in a modified degree, for we still "war" with words, thoughts and feelings over this self-same hypothesis of a "God" and a "Devil."

A careful diagnosis of the disease of the people who go to make up the present metaphysical movement will discover the cause of their particular malady.

The God and devil microbes are quite as much in evidence in the Advanced Thought field as they are in the chronic, hopeless instances of Calvinistic orthodoxy.

The word "sin" is derived from the Hebrew shin, meaning stellar or astral light. The Kabalistic number of Shin (sin) is twenty-one, or three times seven. Twenty-two is the complete number of Hebrew cosmogony, and twenty-one is falling short of completeness by one. "Sin" in Greek also means "falling short" or failure to reach completeness. Unborn millions cannot be saved from failure to comprehend Truth by the crucifixion of a saint.

The New Thought people laugh the orthodox-devil out of court, and then talk much of "error," but just what difference exists between error and "evil" (or devil) is not apparent.

The materialistic concept of the Bible creates many

devils. Evil or a devil of some brand seems an actual necessity to those still in the thought of separateness. The efforts of the evolutionists to keep before the minds of people something other than divine wisdom calls to mind the boy who asked his mother if God would let him have a nice little devil of his own to play with when he went to Heaven if he were real good here.

Some people have such a mania for owning things, as our good Saint Whitman put it, that they say "my catarrh," "my rheumatism," "my cold," etc. Thus, too, do they cherish their "own little devils" and go their way rejoicing in their "very own" complaints.

The modern church took the alchemical and astrological symbols, used by the wise ones of old, clothed them with personalities, prompted by priestly graft, and then called upon everybody to fall down and worship them or go to hell. The Spiritualists, most of them, believe in millions of little evil spirits, but ridicule the orthodox belief in one big evil spirit. Theosophists do not believe in little or big devils—personal—but they do so love their "bad Karma"—the very worst brand of devil in the whole family of devils. Then came Mrs. Eddy with her "mortal mind" devil, occupying a sort of fourth dimension or no place, being a very highly triturated potency of nothing—but a very malignant devil just the same.

The New Thought people having signally failed to get rid of the devil by the philosophy of Spiritualism, Theosophy, or Christian Science, Mental Science, came on the stage to take a hand in the fight. Mental Scientists did not believe in mortal mind. They believed that all was Immortal Mind, or at least they professed to, and it did look for a time as if the devil was really "laid" at last. But upon investigation it was found that the devil had again bobbed up serenely and was doing business at the same old stand, disguised as "Error," "Imperfection," "Mistakes," "Evolution," etc.

The devil in any disguise he may be clothed will continue to give New Thought people trouble.

Of all the negative conditions—devils—the race is subject to, Fear is the greatest. We are born cowards. Our mothers feared for us before we were born. We came into earth-life with a wail of fear. All who had anything to do with us feared something evil would happen to us. They were afraid we would catch cold, or the measles, or whooping cough, or diphtheria, or die of summer complaint. Somebody feared all the time that we would get scalded or frozen, or fall out of bed, or down stairs, or into the well.

When we were old enough to be afraid, we feared our parents, our teachers, the ministers, the dark, the devil, and even feared God, whom St. John says is Love. Later, we were afraid in business, of fire; afraid the election would start some one to tinkering with the tariff, or our blessed money system. We were afraid on land and sea, of fire and water, cold and heat, wind and hail, lightning and cyclone, earthquake and tidal wave, and yet we wonder why there are so many sick people. But the silliest of all fears is the fear of microbes.

We laughed at the elephant because it fears a mouse, but the ignorance of the elephant in that respect is pure wisdom when compared with man's fear of contagious diseases, and his senseless efforts to "stamp them out," by quarantine, disinfectants, germicides, lymphs, serums, and vaccine pus galore.

Paradoxes upon paradoxes! Yet all will cease when competition is supplanted by co-operation. So, then, to sum up, we must find the reason for competition. Man has fostered competition because he thought he was an individual. Man has turned the mighty power he possesses to every obect and principle of force in the universe, except himself, the greatest miracle of all. When man focuses his divine thinking lens upon himself, he will realize that he is an epitome of unlimited Cosmic Energy. Then the "Heavens will roll together as a scroll" and reveal the Real Man as "the Lamb of God that taketh away the sins of the world."

I have seen the surface of flowing rivers changed to ice by the chemical action of cold. I have seen this crystalized water break into countless pieces by the action of heat. I have seen this grotesque, jagged army rush down the great waterways like a charge of cavalry and sweep away iron-girded bridges that an hour before had safely borne the traffic of commercialism. I have seen these huge blocks of ice beat and batter and heard their grinding crash, like the hammer of Thor at the gates of the imperial cities of civilization. I have seen the surface of human thought smooth and petrified by inaction, conversation and respectability. Under the influence of love and wisdom, or in the presence of a great necessity, I have seen this petrification break into projectiles of dynamic thought, dominated with some new concept of life, and hurl themselves against the mailed forces of error and prejudice, until domes and citadels and towers reeled and fell.

As the blocks of ice finally melt and become one, with their primale elements, so will diversity of thought finally unite and blend by the Chemistry of Energy into one harmonious whole.

CONSCIENCE A CREATURE OF EDUCATION.

The Hindu, the Mohammedan, say that their conscience hurts them when they eat meat. Not so with the Christian. The so-called followers of Christ eat the corpses of animals without suffering "Qualms of Conscience."

The concept of right and wrong originates in suggestion, comparison and education.

People generally believe what they are taught in youth. The conscience of the Kaiser caused him to destroy Belgium and plunge Europe into war and he believed that he was God's especial agent.

The different phases of what is known as religion and morals are beliefs based on education. These ideas are simply viewpoints arrived at by comparison or the relation of this to that. Thus the deductions depend upon the scope of the intellect to work and opportunity to obtain data in relation to the matter to be decided.

If conscience was an inward monitor—a Divine Guide —then no one would ever change their opinion or their course in life. The users of tobacco and alcoholic drinks are as conscientious as the abstainers from these poisons; the difference lies in the viewpoint. Thus, "There is nothing right or wrong, but thinking makes it so."

————————

THE COMING MAN.

————

Out of the chemicalizing mass   out of the chemistry of elements, principles, minerals and monads—out of oxygen, hydrogen, nitrogen, carbon, helium, uranium, radium, arum, argentum, potassium sodium and iron— out from these molecules composing the substance of God a new man will be born, a real Son of God who will bear away the sins of the world. I see this form— physical body materializing out of the fomentation of life's creative compounds.

Now hasten vibration from Uranus and vitalize the Etheric Substance that sweeps through the rivers of Eden—the veins and arteries that carry the red cells of omnipresent life. Touch with thy fingers of fire, Golden Haired Apollo, the keys of the new man's won- drous brain until every atom and fiber of the holy temple joins in the Anthem of the stars. And Neptune, thou planet of Realization; at last thy hour has struck. Patient as the Divine Mother thou hast waited for the man.

Lift thy Trident, O Trinity of Life, Liberty and Love, and send to Earth thy pent up vibrations of glory:

Lo; the Aquarius Age;—The new Heaven and new Earth;—

The Co-operative Commonwealth;—The Brotherhood of man.

WHAT DO YOU WANT?

Men, women and children.

Children, women and men—what do they want?

Standing on a street I watched the crowd of men, women and children, some walking fast—some walking slowly—but every face in that endless procession wore the anxious, uncertain look of the aimless.

I attended a lecture; the speaker's subject was "What Do You Want?" The speaker addressed the chairman and then asked of the audience, "What do you want?"

The first to respond was an elderly woman, who arose and said, "I want $150." The speaker then asked, "What do you want $150 for?" The woman replied, "I want the money to buy a horse and buggy." The speaker then replied, "I see by your answer that it is not the money you really want, but a horse and buggy."

But did the woman really want a horse and buggy? No, she wanted some means of travel. If she could have had an automobile, or if some friend had agreed to drive her in another carriage wherever and whenever she wished to ride at less cost than the keep of a horse and buggy, it would have been quite satisfactory.

It was a safe and pleasant conveyance from place to place the woman wanted, but she thought she wanted money.

But there is an occult reason for wanting something. The idea back of every want is a desire for HAPPINESS. No one desires anything that will cause unhappiness, and yet most people are decidedly unhappy. All unhappiness arises from the fact that men and women are slaves to fear. The race is actually in bondage to fear. No one is a slave who is fit for freedom, and no slave can be happy. Freedom, entire freedom from creeds, customs, laws, rules, opinions, threats, belief in evil here or hereafter, and freedom from fear—even the fear of death—is a condition precedent to happiness.

If the above contention is logical, it follows without question that what every human being really wants is freedom. One may say he wants money, or property, or fame, or position, but his only real want is freedom which leads to happiness.

THE FOURTH DIMENSION—VIBRATION—WHAT I SAW AT THE SANTA MONICA SPEEDWAY.

They seemed like great animals, those living, breathing, roaring, snapping auto racers.

I wondered much about the theory of "rates of motion" being the solution of all phenomena. If those who survive the ordeal of the transition from the third to the fourth dimension of space (or whatever it may be) can be accounted good reliable witnesses, the apparent increase of air resistance according to speed does not hold good beyond from 90 to 100 miles per hour.

I saw the winning car plunge forward, the air shrieking about the ears of the driver and mechanician as if it was being tortured on some infernal rack invented by seven times damned spirits, while the earth trembled as if an earthquake was regnant.

As the car swept past round after round, the spaces shriveling up behind it like a tiny bit of bacon on a hot griddle, it seemed to me that the shadowy looking objects directing the flying bolt could not possibly hold their sitting. All seemed uncertain, unsteady and shaky. Then the man with a megaphone roared out, "No. 23 going 72 miles per hour." Another lap, and— "No. 23, 88. Can you beat it?"

Then some one called out, "Look! Here she comes." I looked—or tried to look. There was a flash, like— well, let me think: Did you ever look at a leaf lit up by a ray of sunlight just as a bird's shadow flitted across it? Well, it was something on that order.

And the man with the megaphone called out, "23 going at rate of 97—can you beat it?"

Yes, 23 has just turned the corner half mile north of the grandstand and will pass again—but see! the car and the men seem plain and distinct. Have they slowed down for a stop? No, for they have passed and are now half mile south at the dangerous turn, and while I wondered what caused the firm, solid, steady, unwavering appearance of car and its occupants, he of the megaphone spoke thus: "23 made three-quarters at 105½—can you beat it?"

Here comes 23 again! Now I look closely, intently. I seem to see a sort of opaque substance, impacted ether, or solidified air in front of the car, something that had ceased to resist the car and is now going meteor-like with the great swift animal, No. 23. I could imagine that this impacted ether had by some subtle alchemy detached itself from the fourth dimension, reached forth into the third and drawn the car into its own realm of vibration. But 23 has won, and as it comes down on the last lap the air resistance is again noticeable, the cloud of **something** has dissolved and the car and men wobble like a top that is about to fall over.

THE COMET'S MESSAGE.

I come from the regions of star-dust,
  From the Holies of Infinite Light,
And burn my flaming pathway
  Across the dusk of night.

I hold the keys of Wisdom;
  The keys to the Cosmic Whole,
And offer complete redemption
  To every troubled soul.

I am an electric messenger
  From the outermost circle of space,
And bring Freedom's Manifesto
  To an Earth-bound doubting race—

The message of law eternal,
  Of the Infinite Perfect ways,
The Process forever proceeding
  In the Mind of "The Ancient Days."

I am Perfection's symbol,
  The Apostle of Being Supreme,
The Cosmic Plans Evangel—
  The manifest thought of the "Dream."

I salute the Sentinel Arcturus
  That stands alert and alone,
And cast my rays to Pleiades,
  That wheel around Alcyone.

I rush onward toward Orion,
  The god of the Southern Stars,
And speak a word of Love and Peace
  To the fiery planet Mars.

To Earth, in its throes and Convulsions,
  To Souls struggling up from the Sod,
I bring Brotherhood's Creed plain-worded
  And the Oneness and goodness of God.

I see the world's armies and navies,
  I hear their fierce cries for war,
And trail out my signal: "Peace on Earth"
  From my highway through space afar.

The "Son of Man" cometh in glory,
  His Kingdom will soon appear;
Prepare ye the way for its coming,
  The light of "New Heaven" draws near.

Farewell, I go on my mission;
  When I call on my circle again,
May Earth transmuted and holy,
  Be the Peace habitation of men.
  February, 1909.

BEACHEY.

Birdman! Superman!
  King of the sky.
Thy courage shames our cowardice.
  Goodby, Beachey! Goodby!

Science crowns thee,
  Fame on her scroll
Writes in letters large
  The reward of thy soul.

Thy home the stormclouds,
  The ocean thy bier;
The world loves thee, Beachey,
  While pouring its tears.

On thy spirit airship
  Cleaving the sky—
Goodby, Lincoln Beachey,
  Goodby! Goodby!

THE DAY OF JUDGMENT.

God's loosened thunders shake the world.
Across the lurid sky the war birds scream.
Earth's millions die.
Fear and woe unutterable.
The fires of purification are lighted.
Into the cosmic melting pot has been cast hate, race
    prejudice, selfishness and the devils of greed.
The towers of superstition and tyranny are falling.
The thrones and scepters of kings lie scattered and
    crushed along the highway of nations.
Pride has fallen from its insecure pinnacle of shame.
The rich are terror stricken.
"Their silver has been cast into the street."
"Their gold has been removed from them."

"The merchants of the earth weep and mourn, for no
    man buyeth their merchandise."
The churches are in panic.
The liquor power rages.
The gambler is terror stricken.
The grafting politician seeks a hiding place and finds
    none.
The briber flees when "no man pursueth."
The priest and preacher pray, but no help comes, for
    they too must be judged.
The harlot alone seems unafraid because she is not a
    hypocrite, and has heard the words, "The harlots
    will enter the kingdom before you."
Mankind has gone its limit.
The soul walks forth naked and ashamed.
It is high noon of the Judgment Day.

THE KINGDOM AT HAND.

Man is within one step of his ideal—the ultimate goal
of his desires—that realm of freedom where he will no
longer be subject to law, but being "led by the spirit,"
will realize that he himself is an operator and attribute
of the law.

Man is law in action. Will man now take the final
step into complete liberty and become a god, or continue
to eat of the husks of dual concept and still cower beneath the lash of "precedent and authority?"

There is no "salvation" or regeneration for Man so
long as he believes in vicarious atonement. The man
who needs saving is not worth the price.

Recognition of eternal unity will save Man from the
idea that he needs saving, because it will reconcile him
to his place and mission in the Plan—the Great Neces-

sity. It will reveal to him his true kinship to the cause-less cause, the beginningless beginning, and he will know that he is an attribute of universal energy from which all forms, thoughts, motions, sounds, colors, so-called "good and evil" proceed.

In the full light of this wisdom, Man will not search for saviors nor quibble about the meaning of the words of men who died thousands of years ago.

Christ, Truth, Life—forever preaches the sermon in the ear of Man: "Lo! I am with you now."

Only the spiritually blind look for the "coming" of Truth or Life—the Christ, who is ever present, or the "coming" of a kingdom which is already at hand.

If we accept a certain statement uttered by some one who lived in the dim past, as an ultimatum, we may be called upon to reconcile the utterance with another opin-ion, spoken or written by the same person, which seems to contradict previous statements, in which we have placed our trust.

These persons being dead, cannot be asked for an ex-planation in regard to the seeming contradiction. If they could, they might respond as Walt Whitman did when a critic hinted that the "good gray poet" contradicted him-self: "Do I contradict myself? Then I contradict my-self. I am large, I contain multitudes."

We must consider the facts that the opinions uttered by men in past ages extend over a period of years, dur-ing which time empires rose and fell; new concepts of life obtained recognition due to planetary and zodiacal changes. Thus radical changes occurred in the social, religious, scientific and industrial world.

Viewing the question in this light need we wonder that the seers and sages, saints and scientists of the past should sometimes contradict themselves?

Are we today so very consistent?

Do we not enact what we call "sacred laws," immediately violate them, and carry the case to the court of last resort and get the "sacred" law repealed?

We have had high and low tariff, bimetalism and gold standard, and our great statesmen valiantly upheld the free coinage of silver in the year 1895, and in 1896 these same captains of finance declared through the public press that free coinage of silver would destroy civilization, tear down the pillars of Hercules and wrench the stars from their cosmic thrones.

We have contradicted ourselves in our opinion of the earth's shape, the distance to the Sun, the origin and operation of electricity, the cause of light, the divisibility of elemental gases, the circulation of the blood, the reality of hell and the devil and other subjects too numerous to mention.

Then shall we forever wrangle over the contradictory statements of dead men who wrought in their day as best they might with the light and the data at their command, with no thought that people in future ages would war to the death or live with hate in their hearts for their fellows who differ with them on baptism, the size of Noah's ark, (the moon), or whether a prophet swallowed a fish or a fish swallowed a prophet?

DISEASE NATURE'S EFFORTS TO RESTORE EQUILIBRIUM.

Disease is an alarm signal, a friend that calls to inform us of danger. Disease is an **effort to prevent death**.

Therefore pain and so-called disease is more than a warning; it is an effort that opposes death. The symptoms that indicate disease are calls, or dispatches, asking for the material with which repair of bodily tissue may be made. Pains or discomforts of various functions or structure of the body are **words** asking for the constituent parts of blood, nerve fluids, tissue, bone, etc.

If acids cause pain, the pain is a call for a sufficient amount of alkaloid salts to counteract an acid effect and change fluids to a bland and natural state.

Healthy cynovial fluid (fluids of the joints—the lubricator) is neither acid nor alkali, but yet contains both in combination. Should the alkaline salts become deficient in amount, for any cause, the acid at once becomes a disturbing element and hurts the nerves that pervade the membranes of periosteum (bone covering) of the internal structure of knee, elbow or other joints of the human anatomy. This pain, or word can not be considered bad or malignant in any sense; and to give a Latin or Greek name to this plain demand for lacking material is the insanity of science.

So then it matters not what name may be given to nature's demand for reinforcements through the medium of pain or any symptom that indicates a deviation from the plane of health, **one thing**, and one thing alone is needed, viz.: to supply the blood with the dynamic molecules, the 12 cell-salts, that set up vibration or action in the human machine.

Poisons, of whatever name or nature, do not and cannot supply deficiencies and cure disease for the simple reason that poisons are not constituent parts of the human organism. Poisons oppose calls for help and tend to still the voice of nature; therefore, the effect of poisons is towards death. Many have survived the effect of poisons; but equally many have been hurried to their graves.

A proper use of the mineral, or cell-salts, of the blood in the potency and proportion found in the ashes of a cremated body will do all that can be done medicinally to supply deficiencies and restore normal conditions.

The cell-salts form the chemical base of blood, and blood builds all tissue and fluids of the body.

Anarchy is increasing. A lot of people even refuse to be poisoned by vaccine pus, and some have declared their intention to select their own mode of treatment when sick. Now it is up to the law makers to "stamp out such anarchistic doctrine."

The bacteriologists—may the devil fly away with the whole batch of them—have discovered the kissing microbe and are trying their patent germ killer on it. How fortunate they did not discover and kill that particular germ when our parents were girls and boys.

The second statement in the platform of the Mental Science Association reads: "We maintain that the race is as yet in the infancy of its development, and destined to evolve to infinitely higher standards." And yet there is indubitable proof that a high civilization existed on earth one hundred and fifty thousand years ago.

Back of every dark age the excavator finds indubitable proof of buried civilization and the evolutionist searches in vain for the first "low form of life," saurian or snake, molusk or monkey, from whom he may claim his descent.

There is no reward in the Eternal Plan for doing good, for that which one calls good another calls evil.

All so-called matter is Energy (all there is) in concrete form, or rate of motion.

If men and women are not happier but rather more miserable under the rule of so-called civilization why call the result progression?

Religion has been preached from the pulpit quite long enough. Suppose we set it to work on week days between man and man.

The wise man discovers your good points. The fool sees only your faults.

Eternal life—the only life—operates through the cellular structure of the universe, from the saurian to the savage, from the crystal to the civilizee. A difference in the chemical combination of atoms causes different types of material forms.

No, an acorn does not contain an oak tree, neither does a brick nor a plank contain a house. The acorn is a bit of concentrated oxygen, hydrogen, carbon, mineral salts, etc. It is the beginning of an oak tree just as a brick, board or stone may be the commencement of a house. As it requires more boards or bricks to build a house, so does it require more of the constituents of a tree—elements in the acorn—to build a tree.

Neither books, nor prophets, nor bibles, nor saints, nor sages, nor saviors make Truth.

Truth is eternal. It liveth forevermore.

Go not into the desert nor to the mountain top to find thy ideal—for "Lo!" the kingdom of Heaven is at hand."

Morality can not be put into the Alembic and reduced to its constituent parts. That which is lawful, and therefore moral, in Turkey may be unlawful and immoral in other countries.

The Christian dines on the corpses of animals, fishes and fowls, while the Buddhist revolts at the feast of flesh and declares the practice not only immoral but also criminal.

Right and wrong seem to be largely determined by georgraphy.

A dog is none the less a nuisance because he wears a silver collar, neither is the innate character of man changed one whit by a gilded badge of distinction.

All phenomena appears as a result of Divine, beneficent law, hence disease so-called is the result of the orderly proceedure of that law. In all ages all men and women have been sick more or less. In all ages there have been storms, cataclysms, earthquakes and extremes of heat and cold; no one questions the wisdom that causes, guides and directs these events, then why should we question the wisdom of disease? Disease is one phase of transmutation of matter in the proceedure of regeneration.

All methods of healing are phases of the transmutation process.

When man reaches the plane of understanding (Alchemical Knowledge) he will consciously co-operate with the Divine Urge by supplying his dynamic laboratory with the mineral base of blood (the Philosopher Stone), and thus make blood the "Elixir of Life" as it is destined to be.

Consider Biochemistry, thou invalid, study her truths, practice her precepts and you will not only obtain wisdom, but you will also realize that you are a worker in the plan of regeneration.

The Co-operative Commonwealth will appear when real red blood fills the veins and arteries of men and women.

LINCOLN.

He struck the flint of prejudice and old tradition with the steel of truth until the sparks of freedom lighted the dark abyss of error. He wrote the autograph of brotherhood across the nation's scroll—then lifted his stalwart arm and struck the shackels from the slave.

EDISON.

He sports with nature's forces as a child plays with toys; brings forth from throats of brass with fingers of steel the notes of music that once ran riot through a singer's brain; splits cosmic stuff into atoms, ions, electrons—then touches them with some magic brain-wand of genius until like concentrated intelligence they spring from carbon crucible, illuminate our homes and streets, set awhir the machinery of the world, o'erleaps desert

sands and snarling seas and cries aloud: "Lo, here am
I!"

WALT WHITMAN.

A god-made flesh appeared—wrote some words on
paper and then retired to his abode behind the veil.

After many years a few, in their Great Adventure,
on the road to liberty dared to read the words written
by the god. Some understood and found the land of
"heart's desire"—the freedom of the mind.

EMERSON.

The musician of the soul. He who came and touched
a chord of the human harp, so long unused that e'er its
tones came forth to thrill the heart, the Harper had
departed on his way. And even now we must tiptoe and
hold back the breath to catch even faint echoes from
that smitten chord that shall forevermore vibrate with
the music of the stars.

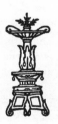

It is only by forgiving one's self and realizing perfection in the here and now that we can realize the full meaning of the proverb, "Charity begins at home." Again, "Love thy neighbor as thyself" is literally obeyed by everybody. So long as one believes himself imperfect or criticises himself he will criticise his neighbor. Man really loves his neighbor as himself, but his love is a kind that makes the angels weep. When a man really loves himself—sees himself as a divine attribute—his love for his neighbor will make angels smile.

Earth is one of the heavenly planets and there is not a grain of evidence that any other planet or world is any better than Earth; nor is there any reason to think that we can be happier or more contented in any other world than we can be here.

Until man can know what a bird, reptile or beast thinks and knows, he can not say he knows more than they. The idea of lower forms of life is an egotistic concept based in dense ignorance. I am tired of hearing it said that man is the highest expression of life. Why bless your soul, man can neither fly like a bird, live in water like a fish nor materialize air like a spider.

"Thinking he is a mistake and the universe a hotchpotch man criticises himself, and criticises his neighbors as himself, which makes angels weep.

When man realizes that he is an attribute of Perfect Law he will love himself because he will love the law; and he will love his neighbor as he loves himself and the law.

_____

SHAKESPEARE.

He struck the Camp of Knowledge on the road of

Man's Desire centuries beyond his time and rationed it with food for countless men unborn.

He probed the deeps of human possibilities, analyzed the stuff from which thoughts are made, turned the searchlight of incomparable genius on the records of the soul, painted its deeds on the canvas of life and left it naked and ashamed.

HUMANITY'S CEASELESS QUEST FOR THE END OF THE LONG ROAD.

The child asked its parents, "Where does the road end?" and was told that the road entered another road and that that road entered another road and so on, forever. But the child was not satisfied. The boy asked his schoolmates where the road ended and they answered, "This road runs down by the mill and enters the road to the village, and the road there enters the big road that goes away to the west."

The young man asked his college chums, "Where does the road end that runs toward the west?" and they answered, "We do not know; maybe there is no end."

The young man soon realized that his chums were not interested about the end of the road. They liked games and sports and moonlight boating on the lake with their sweethearts. The man entered into business; he bought and sold for profit; he collected rents; he loaned money at interest; he became wealthy."

The man asked the members of his firm, "Where does the road end?" His business associates were engrossed in trade, in stocks and bonds, and had never given a thought about the end of the road.

The man passed middle age, grew tired of the grind of commercial life and entered the political arena. He saw honor bought and sold like merchandise. He assisted in framing laws and assisted in repealing the laws. He grew weary of the treadmill of politics and asked the lawyers and judges, "Where does the road end?" The judges and lawyers looked wise, but could not answer. They did not know where the road ended.

The man retired from politics and joined an exclusive club. He rested for hours in luxurious apartments. He read books, magazines and newspapers. He attended scientific lectures, but he did not receive any information about the end of the road. Everything that men and women did as they journeyed on the road was done for profit in order that they might have. And the man grew very tired and wished to find the end of the road. The man was old and now cared for but one thing: to find the end of the road. And so he traveled westward.

> "West to the Sinking Sun,
>   Where the junk sails lift
>   In the homeless drift
>   And the East and the West are one."

The old man met many people and asked, "Where does the road end?" but they saw he was old and "childish" and they did not answer. They did not know where the road ended.

The old man was weak and tired and sat down on a mountainside and looked into the west. He saw the shimmer of the Balboa sea and said, "Now I will find the end of the road." And he walked slowly on. He felt the cool breeze of the "sundown sea." He reclined on the sand near the tide line where the spray bathed his face.

The sun was "dipping its forehead in the foam" out in the golden west, and the reflection against the cloudlets looked like a garden of roses in the heavens.

The old man said: "I have found the end of the road," and repeated the lines:

> "Glimmering waters and breakers
> Far on the horizon's rim,
> White sails and sea gulls glinting
> Away 'till the sight grows dim—
> And shells spirit-painted with glory
> Where sea-weeds beckon and nod—
> Some people call it Ocean
> And others call it God."

The waves lapped at the feet of the old man. The sea gulls circled round uttering plaintive cries, and the traveler slept.

"Then the great sun died, and a rose-red bloom grew over his grave in a border of gold.

"And a cloud with a silver rim was rolled like a great gray stone at the door of the tomb."

MOTORMAN! MY MOTORMAN!

> On the edge of the cliff,
> 'Round the danger curve
> I sit and wonder
> At thy hand of nerve—
> Motorman! my motorman!

By the sea-gulls' home
On the crest of the foam
And adown the track
As the waves rush back
Motorman! my motorman!

There's a thought in my soul
"Will he reach the goal"
As he turns headlight
To the mountain height—
Motorman! my motorman!

Then up to the peaks
Where the eagles shriek
We join the strain
The glad refrain—
Motorman! my motorman!

When the moon-mad sea
Sends its tide for me
To the other shore
Oh then once more
Motorman! my motorman!

He who sacrifices more for another than he would be willing to accept under like conditions is not treating himself justly.

A literal interpretation of the mythological characters, astronomical allegories and alchemical symbols of the Bible and New Testament has caused the earth to run red with wars; and the belief that the literal blood of a man, however good, or his ignominious death could by any possibility save souls, has made idolators of a large portion of the race. It seems incredible that men should go to war about God or religion, yet such is the case.

All scripture is an allegory. It is a figurative literality. It described literal facts under the figure of living beings. It is a personification of existing active principles, but no person or sentient thing is actually alluded to from Genesis to Revelations.

To establish this proposition, you say, will subvert all existing religious belief. Not so. It will simply give to religion what it lacks—a scientific and reasonable basis. It will bring the present church out of the crumbling shadows of doubt into the strong light of faith, establishing it upon the rock of eternal truth or science.

The word Satan is from the Sanscrit, Satya, meaning truth, and the Egyptian Soterim, i. e., a judge. It is also identified with the Greek Cronus, meaning one crowned.

The devil is only God in disguise. Spell devil backward and you have "lived"—that is, life, and life is God. Therefore God spelled backward—that is, "lived" —is a combination of letters that spells devil.

Be free, oh soul! Arise, take up thy bed and walk. Thy sins be forgiven thee.

The resurrection morn has dawned. This is the day of judgment; that is, correct judgment.

Men and women are about as happy, or miserable, as they are capable of being. Environments cut little figure in the human drama.

Bunyan wrote a great alegorical book while in prison. Harriet Beecher Stowe wrote a manuscript so terrific in dynamic force that it split the idol of chattel slavery into fragments, even as the lightning shatters a pine, while attending to six children and doing cooking, sewing and general housework.

What shall it profit a man to become an oil king and then flee to Europe to escape the penalty of the laws enacted by his own legislatures and Congress?

Patience is the savior of the world. Astrology teaches patience.

If Mental Scientists will study the writings of Epictitus they will discover that their science was taught more than 4000 years ago.

The Sorrows of Satan are coming hot and heavy. The meat (corpse) trust has made the devil look like 15c at a lunch counter.

The average Mr. Man would rather argue than listen, rather deny than think.

<hr>

MIRACLES.

"I know of nothing but miracles."
—Walt Whitman.

Why search for the miraculous?

The wisdom of the ant or beaver strikes dumb all the believers in the Darwinian dream.

The modus operandi by which a spider materializes its web from air without ever having attended a school of chemistry is the despair of science.

The perfect co-operative commonwealth of the bees is still the dream of man.

Behold the miracle of a bud, a flower; a decaying grain of corn and the thousand grained full ear, burnished with gold and filled with nutriment.

A splendid man and woman today in a home, next

year there are three—a miracle—a babe; forth from the wondrous mother laboratory come the child. The mysteries of conception and birth are miracles.

Man cannot control the growth of his hair or fingernails, and he knows nothing about the process of digestion and assimilation of food.

Miracles! See the brush of Cosmic Law paint the rainbow. Look at a pendant icicle, a drop of dew or a wreath of mist. Observe the clean-trunked eucalypti, the orange blossom, the cactus. See the uprising clouds of morning sprinkling jewels on grass and flowers. Listen to the shuttle threated mocking bird flinging liquid melody into the ears of Deity.

The alchemical operations of a spider puzzles the chemist; and the handiwork of a beaver breaks the spell of the Darwinian dream.

Principle is not changed because this or that has been written about it and printed in a book.

Nothing can be made right or wrong by legal enactments.

Principles are eternal verities, or truths, and therefore not subject to the whims and changes of human laws or statutes.

Each Legislature or Congress repeals and sets at naught the so-called sacred laws of former law-making bodies. Thus do they render null and void one counterfeit by putting into circulation another counterfeit composed of the same base metal bearing a different inscription.

Law cannot be made; it eternally exists; its name is Wisdom, or God, and patient as the sea waits for recognition.

A monkey may be taught to act nearly like a man; but a man often acts like a monkey without the assistance of a teacher.

When we so signally fail to decide what is best for ourselves how shall we advise others.

The birds are beginning to believe in evolution. Since the advent of the Wright Brothers and Count Zeppelin I heard a mocking-bird say, the other day, that it really believed that man could evolute up to the plane of birds within another century.

The Pharaohs of capital are fearful that the Israelites of labor are about to start out for the desert and Red Sea and leave the Napoleons of finance to do their own work.

If Moses would only appear!

It has been discovered that there is a much larger per cent of bribery, defalcation and general dishonesty among bankers and "business men" than among working-men, trades unions and walking delegates. "Comparisons are odious"—to the business man.

The bad man is the man you dislike or who professes a different religion or does that which you do not do.

The ignorant man is one who does not speak your language.

————

Some people have such a "mania for owning things," as good Saint Whitman wrote it, that they say "my catarrh," or "my rheumatism." Thus do they cherish their little devils and go on their way complaining and lamenting.

THE CATACLYSM, 1916.

The dry leaves whirl and swirl,
  And seek a safe retreat,
As sudden gusts blow swift
  Along the dusty road and street.
The frightened moon hides crescent horns
  Behind the hurrying cloud
And vapors dark with border red
  Wraps nature like a shroud.

The seed once sown by selfishness
  Has blossomed in its bed.
The fruit is growing, ripening fast—
  Its color crimson red.
The upas tree bears poisonous fruit,
  Life withers 'neath its shade,
And those who plant and nourish it
  Beneath it shall be laid.

The storm has burst; the cannons roar;
  The earth runs red with blood;
Is this thy peace, O optimist—
  Thy dream of brotherhood?
Shall competition, hate and strife
  And war's dread carnage
Forever write its autograph
  On history's crimson page?

Arise, O man! O woman great!
  And unity thy cry,
Unfurl co-operation's flag,
  And let it wave on high;
And let the new earth onward wheel
  Toward the blessed goal,
And let the new Heaven's choir chant
  The "Triumph of the Soul."

THE IROQUOIS THEATRE TRAGEDY.

"Oh! see the calcium light," they said,
They looked, and then "six hundred dead."

A Simoon wind and fiery dust—
And then the awful holocaust.

From hell a scorching sheet of flame—
And then charred bodies without name.

"Give dividends," the Shylocks cried,
And then six hundred victims died.

But Justice stands with balanced sword
And waits the inevitable word.

Though heaven falls and suns grow dim,
Stern Justice meted out by Him

Who rules the stars—shall never cease
Until on earth the reign of Peace.

———————

This, strictly private—just for you and I: We are
immersed in the universal energy from which all forms
or manifestations proceed. What more can we ask?

———

We are operators of the Divine, or Cosmic machine.
Suppose that you and I try to become conscious of the
mighty truth.

———————

A SONG OF PEACE.

———

The stars in their course
Are nearing the dawn of peace.
The purpling mountain tops
Of human love appear.
Look! Listen!
Above the battle's din you may hear
The anthem of "Peace on earth."
Good will to men is in the air.

Out from the curling mists of the Pacific sea,
That twist and twine
Like things alive.
From the glory of the up-climbing clouds
Of the morning that spill their jewels
On the grass and flowers.
In the liquid notes of the shuttle-throated mocking bird
That pours its rippling prayers
Into the ears of Deity.

From the clean-trunked eucalypti,
From orange blossoms and pendant pepper bough.
From the sweet-faced little children,
From the hearts of earnest men,
From the souls of women's mothers,
From the planetary angles
And rising constellations.

From the heavenly hosts that
"Declare the glory of God,"
From the inner sanctuary of cosmic law—
We may hear the song of Peace.
Peace comes!
Reach forth thy hands, brothers, sisters,
Welcome thy Savior—Peace.

Flowers bloom fresh in her footsteps;
The folds of her white garments are like "trailing clouds
　　　of glory."
The co-operative commonwealth of humanity looms be-

hind her.
The bugles all sing truce along the iron front of war.

Offend her not.
Bow to the radiant queen.
We are so weary—
Yea, sick unto death—of war.
Our Healer comes—
The Great Physician.
Let all rejoice and be glad.
Let us join the song, Peace Unto Thee.

Behold the new earth.
Ironclads rust.
The trenches are covered with grass.
Vines clamber over arsenals.
Flowers bloom on deserted forts.
Soldiers become men, at home, field, shop, firesides.
Women love and children play.
"The ransomed of the Lord return
And come to Zion—
With everlasting joy upon their heads."
And all over and about
The air is full of the scent of flowers
And the trickling fall of fountains,
And free souls have started on the
Great Adventure
To find God.

And thus the "last enemy has been overcome" and
death destroyed by the realization of Abundant Life.

This is the Resurrection Morn—the Day of Judgment. The "New Heaven and New Earth" has appeared.
The Angel Choir chants "Peace on Earth, Good Will to
Men," and mankind, awakened and redeemed, joins in
the anthem of the Heavenly Host.

ETHER; OR, THE IMPOSSIBLE.

Written by an Insane Man.

I met an impossible man, and this is what he said: "Nothing but the impossible is true. The possible is too easy to be true. The possible is a fleeting illusion of the senses. The impossible is the solid, immovable, concrete uni verse. It is immovable because there is no room for movement or vibration.

So, then, everything that the possible man thinks is possible, namely, substance, motion, etc., is an illusion; and that which he thinks is impossible, namely, a solid statu quo verse, without motion, life or intelligence, or any other known quality, is the only truth.

Thought, the impossible thing, being no thing, operates on or in this impossible verse or crystal deadness, and paints transitory figures mathematical, geometrical, algebraical, geographical, chemical and alchemical.

Impossible no thing, called thought, or ether, thus gives expression to its nonenity in order to realize something.

The rapidly changing films of a moving picture machine is the nearest approach of an illustration of the impossible, yet attained on or in the solid impossible crystal-mirror-globe, or universe. Being one, there can be no thing between the molecules or atoms—yea, there cannot be any such things as atoms or molecules in One Verse.

The singular is not composed of things. It is not composed at all. Being one, proves that it is no thing, therefore impossible, therefore True.

The word possibility indicates doubt, which is prima

facie evidence of fraud, and fraud vitiates everything that it touches, proving the contention that everything that is possible-ity has been destroyed, leaving only the impossible no-thing which cannot be contaminated and which, therefore, is true.

Man's body, and other so-called objects, seem to move. One who did not know would say they were living moving bodies on the stage in the moving picture show. All there is of the picture is thought behind the manifestation. Man's body is a picture, or appearance painted by nonentity thought on the solid, immovable, impossible, crystal, concrete sea of stuff that is unnamable. Yet we may call it the frozen mathematical formulae that symbols God.

All that I have written is easily proven to one illumined. It is foolishnes only to a fool."

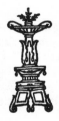

Press of the "Astrological Bulletina" monthly magazine. Box 638, Portland, Oregon.

ZODIACAL CELL-FOODS

★

FOR YOUR HEALTH

The "Grand Man" of the zodiac, which is usually illustrated in the common almanacs, is said to be the work of Hippocrates, who was a famous Greek physician popularly called "The Father of Medicine," and who said, "A physician cannot safely administer medicine if he be unacquainted with Astrology."

The body of the "Grand Man" has been divided into 12 zones, each part represented by a Sign of the Zodiac, beginning with Aries, the head, and proceeding down to Pisces, the feet. Persons born in the month of a Sign ruling a certain part of the body are usually susceptible to disorders in that part. Having greater cellular activity there they usually become deficient in the salts of the blood which particularly supply that part. Hence, people are often greatly benefited by partaking of the Zodiacal Cell Foods corresponding to their birth month sign, in addition to the Cell-Foods. they may need for particular ailments.

The human body is a vessel of liquid (being seven-tenths fluidic) and subtle chemicals, which are readily affected by planetary currents, indeed. the metabolism of the body owes its direction largely to planetary influence. Waves of light, heat and sound also effect it, in accordance with the position of the Sun and planets at the time of birth.

One of the world's great philosophers said, "if, as we know, the planets have an influence upon the earth's magnetic and physical currents, then the conclusion is irresistible that they must have an influence upon mankind, for man is but an atom or particle of an harmonious whole. He partakes of every element of the universe, and is, therefor, subject to the grand laws of eternal and immutable harmony."

If we wish to make the most of our life and derive the greatest benefits as the result of our endeavors, we needs must understand nature's laws and work consciously in harmony therewith. The Divine plan did not create human beings for a life of suffering, misery and disease; these are the results of lack of understanding and cooperation with the creative principles of nature, but such difficulties can be corrected by proper effort.

Our forefathers lived to a hearty and vigorous old age—why is the present generation so short-lived? Largely because of the artificial conditions in which we live. Our foods no longer contain enough of the vital elements which are so essential to the growth, repair and perpetuation of the bodily structure and detrioration is the result. The nerve force is weakened and the blood supply deficient through the starvation engendered by adulterated foods, watered milk, polished rice, white bread, etc., etc.

Our forefathers were "hardy" largely because the foods they ate were from virgin soil, rich in the natural salts which go to sustain life in a healthy manner—consequently, they were better nourished than men of today whose food is largely obtained from worn-out and unscientifically nurtured soil, in addition to the lamentable fact that crops are planted and plucked haphazardly, instead of being planted and gathered in the proper zodiacal signs, for, when properly planted, they produce larger quantities of life-sustaining cell salt foods.

The human organism needs an adequate supply of lime, iron, sulphur, magnesia, silica, potash, soda, sulphates, phosphates and chlorates—12 principal life sustaining elements. When a deficiency of one of these salts occurs the functions served by that salt fall below par, leading to dis-ease and dis-organization. The science of Biochemistry supplies such deficiencies by providing 12 especially prepared Cell Salts named after the Signs of the Zodiac because of their effect upon the corelated organs and functions of the 12 zones in the body.

When the earth becomes "worn out" by continuous crops the land must be fertilized by the application of phosphate or lime, etc.; ground that is used must be fed, its deficiencies must be supplied, else it becomes valueless.

The human body to be kept in a healthy condition must be supplied with the needed Salts. Many farmers are aware that lime will "sweeten" the soil and prevent worms from working around the trees, and that it will add a bright, luxuriant appearance to foliage. In the human body it has been found that a deficiency of the element which lime supplies to the blood causes fermentation, belching and acid conditions to arise. A deficiency of lime also permits the breeding of worms, decay of teeth, and a weakness in the bony structure. In parts of the country where the drinking water is notably deficient in lime, unsound teeth are prevalent.

It has been found in the cases where children are small, weak, nervous, bow-legged, sickly and who suffer greatly from teething, that some form of lime administered will supply the deficiency in the system and they soon become healthy, strong, normal children. Lime is a Capricorn Salt; Capricorn is ruled by Saturn; throughout all ages, it has been known that Saturn rules the bones and teeth. It is known that where the drinking water is hard, where the soil is rich in lime and magensia, teeth are free from decay.

When Saturn is afflicted at the time of someone's birth, that person will be deficient in lime and will manifest the defect by the above symptoms in childhood, and throughout all their life they need lime or they will be insufficiently nourished and suffer accordingly, regardless of whether or not they were born in the month of Capricorn, i. e., between December 22nd and January 19th, any year.

As stated previously—people are usually deficient in the Cell Salts corresponding to their birth sign and the sign Ascending at birth. For instance, an Astrological text book (A to Z Horoscope Delineator in part IV) gives the following description of a person with Capricorn as their Ascending Sign: "Stature is average to short; generally defective walk and a liability to rheumatism in the joints, or marks and scars about the knees; usually they are thin and bony; prominent features, usually long and thin; long or prominent nose; thin neck; long chin; hair dark or black, not over plentiful; thin beard; usually not handsome."

Remember that Saturn rules the Sign Capricorn; Saturn rules lime; the above description in Astrology would signify in Biochemistry a deficiency in lime or the Capricorn Cell Food.

In other words, the metabolism of the body usually uses up the salts of the ascending or birth month signs faster than it uses the salts of other signs and therefore requires fortification with frequent administration of those particular Cell Foods.

Not only does a deficiency in some Cell Foods affect the body but also the mind and moral tendencies, producing some degree of perversion according to its nature. The effect of a deficiency in lime tends to mental states of timidity, fear, nervousness, depression, lack of optimism, and inclines one to be skeptical, deceitful, exacting, avaricious, perverse, indifferent, laborious, impotent, acquisitive, secretive, suspicious, slow, callous, lewd, with periods of inertia and vitiated feelings.

The foregoing is an exact description of an afflicted Saturn affecting the mental activities. (A to Z Horoscope Delineator, Chapter 1, Planetary Natures and Correspondence). When planets affect the body adversely, the science of Biochemistry offers the means of correcting the conditions.

There are three forms of lime, designated as Capricorn, Scorpio and Cancer Salts. A lack of the Scorpio Salts in the system produces the effects known as bronchitis, lung disease, boils, carbuncle, ulcers, abscesses, advanced stage of catarrh, or exudations from any part of the body. The action of Scorpio Salt is opposite to the action of the Sagittarius Salt; Sagittarius hastens the process of suppuration while Scorpio closes up a process that has continued too long. A deficiency of the Cancer Salt causes a relaxed condition of muscular tissue, prolapsus of uterus, varicose veins, swellings of stony hardness. Frequently it produces groundless fears of financial ruin.

A deficiency of the Virgo Salt (Sulphate of Potash) causes a clogging of the pores through a disturbance in the distribution of oil in the system causing oily, slimy, yellowish exudations from any orifice of the body, or from any glandular swellings, abscesses, cancers. etc.: likewise. dandruff or eruptions and falling out of hair.

Many of the noted mineral springs owe their reputation for cures to the Silica (Sagittarius Salt) held in solution in their waters, because people who were lacking in Silica were benefited thereby, whereas, many people who have visited springs were not benefited because they were not deficient in the Salts furnished by that spring. Mineral springs furnish certain salts and will benefit people needing those salts.

The human body being composed of two kinds of matter, organic and inorganic, neither of which can perform its functions without the other, requires that they be kept in harmonious and well balanced relation, to produce the best expression of a healthy life. Oxygen carbon, sulphur, iron, phosphorus, chlorine, fluorine, silicon, magnesia, sodium, calcium and potassium are the elements which the blood relies on principally, to feed and nourish the body. When any of these are lacking certain cells are starved and cannot perform their function—dis-ease is the result—supply the deficiency and the cause of the disease is removed.

A plant will droop for the want of water, or proper fertilizing material, phosphate, lime, potash, etc., which are constituent parts of the plant and absolutely necessary for its healthy growth. The human body, much more highly complex in its organism, will droop if deficiencies occur in the functional necessities. To restore and maintain the body in a healthy condition by supplying the necessary elements, is the mission of Biochemistry. Nature is the healer but it must have the necessary elements with which to exercise its healing powers. Sometimes these elements are created by the vibration caused by the laying of hands upon afflicted parts; sometimes by strong, well directed thought currents; sometimes by ardent prayer, but Biochemistry aims to supply deficiencies through use of the 12 principal Cell Foods.

Physicians of the early days—of the school of Hippocraties, "the father of medicine," understood the administration of herbs ruled by the signs of the zodiac. Our grandfathers also gathered herbs, roots, barks, berries and plants according to the signs of the zodiac during the proper seasons of the year, so that they could assist nature in overcoming the different ailments which might occur. But through the science of Biochemistry the salts are obtained in more reliable potencies and in their pure crystal state through the processes of precipitation, to be used singly or in groups, as may be seen fit, without causing weakened digestive organs the laborious process of extracting them from the unpleasant foreign matter contained in many plants.

Biochemic Zodical Cell Foods are pleasant and palatable, being presented in convenient tablet form which readily dissolve on the tongue, entering the system in a state ready for immediate assimilation.

Self treatment by means of the Biochemic Foods is rapidly becoming a popular means of overcoming bodily disorders. Thousands of people testify to the favorable results obtained. A fair trail will convince any one of their efficacy.

Because of our belief in the value of Cell Foods we are acting as General Agents for their distribution.

"Cell Foods"

"Cell Foods" are the 12 Biochemic Salts, each named after the Sign of the Zodiac to which it corresponds. We carry in stock a supply of each of the 12 "Cell Foods," any kind of which may be purchased from us at $1.00 per box, sent postpaid. Six boxes for $5.00

Read the circular which describes the virtues of each of the twelve "Cell Foods" from Aries, No. 1, to Pisces. No. 12. Two or more kinds of "Cell Foods" can be used by taking alternately.

We do not prescribe. Read the description of the 12 "Cell Foods" and choose those which are best suited to your needs.

Note the books which are given **free** with $3.00 or or $5.00 orders *IF REQUESTED.*

"The twelve Cell Salts and the Zodiac," given free, upon request, with $3.00 orders.

"Biochemic Pathology of Disease," given **free**, upon request, with $5.00 orders.

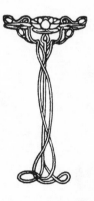

General Agents for Cell Foods
THE LLEWELLYN PUBLISHING CO.
1507 S. Ardmore Ave., Los Angeles, California.

CPSIA information can be obtained
at www.ICGtesting.com
Printed in the USA
LVHW041301090520
655281LV00003B/963